MY POCKET MENTOR: A HEALTH CARE PROFESSIONAL'S GUIDE TO SUCCESS

Sandra Gaviola

THOMSON

DELMAR LEARNING   Australia   Canada   Mexico   Singapore   Spain   United Kingdom   United States

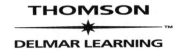

THOMSON

DELMAR LEARNING

My Pocket Mentor: A Health Care Professional's Guide to Success

By Sandra Gaviola

Vice President,
Health Care Business Unit:
William Brottmiller

Executive Director:
Cathy L. Esperti

Acquisitions Editor:
Marah Bellegarde

Developmental Editor:
Debra Flis

Editorial Assistant:
Erin Adams

Marketing Director:
Jennifer McAvey

Marketing Channel Manager:
Tamara Caruso

Production Editor:
Anne Sherman

COPYRIGHT © 2004 by Delmar Learning, a division of Thomson Learning, Inc.
Thomson Learning™ is a trademark used herein under license.

Printed in Canada
2 3 4 5 XXX 08 07 06

For more information, contact Delmar Learning, 5 Maxwell Drive, Clifton Park, NY 12065
Or find us on the World Wide Web at http://www.delmarlearning.com

ALL RIGHTS RESERVED. 2005, 1999. No part of this work covered by the copyright hereon may be reproduced or used in any form or by any means—graphic, electronic, or mechanical, including photocopying, recording, taping, Web distribution or information storage and retrieval systems—without written permission of the publisher.
For permission to use material from this text or product, contact us by
Tel   (800) 730-2214
Fax   (800) 730-2215
www.thomsonrights.com

Library of Congress Cataloging-in-Publication Data

My pocket mentor : a health care professional's guide to success / Sandra Gaviola . . . [et al.].
      p. ; cm.
Includes bibliographical references and index.
ISBN-13: 978-1-4018-3508-8
ISBN-10: 1-4018-3508-2
1. Allied health personnel—Vocational guidance.
2. Paramedical education. [DNLM:
1. Allied Health Personnel.
2. Vocational Guidance.
3. Professional Role. W 21.5 M995 2005] I. Gaviola, Sandra.   II. Title.

R697.A4M9 2005
610.73'7069—dc22

                                    2003064613

NOTICE TO THE READER

C O N T E N T S

P R E F A C E

This text was written with your personal and professional needs in mind. The authors of *My Pocket Mentor* have prepared a text of virtual do's and don'ts for *you,* the entry-level allied health care student. This text presents easy-to-understand information on a number of practical elements that contribute to your becoming a true professional. Without this information, you can easily and unwittingly slip into a few pitfalls even before your career has taken flight.

The text is prepared in a manner that corresponds with a typical allied health care course curriculum. Chapters 1 through 4 are intended for use in the classroom. In Chapter 1 you will be assured that enrolling in a higher education program requires adjustments and patience. You are reminded that you are not alone and given tips on how to stay motivated and focused. Chapter 2 provides the "inside scoop" from an educator who is certainly on your side. In this chapter you will find help in communicating effectively and professionally with your instructors or professors, establishing a rapport that is highly conducive to learning. We are certain that at one point you will have to prepare a technical paper. The author of Chapter 3, a professional writer, gives her secrets for a satisfying and rewarding writing assignment. And finally, the one lesson that was the inspiration for *My Pocket Mentor:* Chapter 4. This chapter presents the traits that are consistently found in role-model students and employees. You are asked to examine your strengths and weaknesses and identify areas in which you would like to and believe you can improve. This chapter offers invaluable information that will benefit you beyond your role as a student.

Chapter 5 is going to get you off on the right foot as a public speaker. As a health care provider, you accept the ongoing challenge of effective oral communication. Your audience may be a single client or patient or a much larger group of individuals attending a community awareness program or a conference. This chapter will explain the importance of knowing yourself as well as your audience, no matter what size.

If your enthusiasm has waned a bit since the first day of school, don't be discouraged or surprised. Enthusiasm rises and falls throughout life. Chapter 6 describes enthusiasm and how it can be rekindled if you believe you have lost it.

You will find the final four chapters most helpful as you enter the clinical environment. Professional appearance and behavior has changed over the years. The author of Chapter 7 has yet to take her finger off the pulse of professional dress and behavior. Her inclusion of guidelines for body piercings and other forms of body art in the clinical setting is proof of that. Once you are working in the real world, your attentiveness to the client's or patient's needs as well as your accuracy in documenting and communicating with other members of the team will be tested. Chapter 8 will heighten your awareness of a client's or patient's rights as well as special circumstances that must be handled during the interviewing process.

Finally, we are concerned about your needs. Although we cannot predict your resilience, the authors of this text expect that any individual entering the health care profession will experience stressful events. There are smart ways to cope. It would be unfortunate for you if you neglected your health or developed harmful habits in order to deal with stress. Chapter 9 is all about you. Chapter 10 is all about your financial health. Learn from others' mistakes as you read about money management.

The style of communication may vary somewhat from author to author, but we are one voice with one goal . . . your success!

EXTENSIVE TEACHING PACKAGE

An extensive teaching package is available to supplement this book.

Instructor's Manual to Accompany My Pocket Mentor: A Health Care Professional's Guide to Success

The instructor's manual offers additional tools for instructors, including critical thinking exercises, topics for discussion, and personal development experiments. (ISBN 1-4018-3510-4)

Career Success for Health Care Professionals Video Series

This video series takes viewers through all the softskills necessary for personal development and career success. Softskills are skills relating to people issues that include such key concepts as:

- compassion for patients and their circumstances
- verbal and nonverbal communication with patients and within a health care team
- professionalism through appearance, personal hygiene, and vocabulary
- thinking like a health care worker through problem-solving skills
- cooperation within the team and patients and their families

Modeling is an effective way to teach these skills. Realistic behaviors presented in realistic settings and supported by clear commentary and graphic devices help reinforce these concepts. Observing diverse characters in real-life scenarios will best prepare viewers to recognize and anticipate similar communication opportunities in their own lives.

Career Success for Health Care Professionals Video Series (6 tapes)
—ISBN 1-4018-3498-1

Individual Tapes are also available:
  Video 1 Focusing on the Patient (ISBN 1-4018-3499-X)
  Video 2 Communicating on the Job (ISBN 1-4018-3500-7)
  Video 3 Thinking Like a Health Care Worker
      (ISBN 1-4018-3501-5)
  Video 4 Doing the Right Thing (ISBN 1-4018-3503-1)
  Video 5 Achieving Professional Success (ISBN 1-4018-3505-8)
  Video 6 Getting a Job in Health Care (ISBN 1-4018-3506-6)

Instructor's Manual to Accompany Career Success for Health Care Professionals Video Series

The instructor's manual shows how to incorporate the video series into an existing curriculum, how to use the video series as a separate seminar, and how to incorporate other Delmar Learning products to develop a six-week or one-credit hour course. (ISBN 1-4018-3507-4)

Workbook to Accompany Career Success for Health Care Professionals Video Series

The workbook includes pre-tests, exercises, and post-tests for every video to help reinforce concepts. (ISBN 1-4018-3511-2)

A C K N O W L E D G M E N T S

The authors and Delmar Learning would like to thank the following individuals for their valuable feedback:

Marilyn C. Handley, RN, PhD
Assistant Professor
University of Alabama Capstone College of Nursing
McCalla, AL

Judith W. Herrman, RN, PhD
Undergraduate Clinical Coordinator
Department of Nursing
University of Delaware
Newark, DE

Laura Logan, RN, BSN
Program Coordinator for Health Programs
Angelina College
Lufkin, TX

Nancy McGowan, RN, PhD
Assistant Professor
The University of Texas Health Science Center
    at San Antonio
School of Nursing
San Antonio, TX

CONTRIBUTORS

Dianne A. Adams, MA, RRT
Program Administrator
Northwest New Jersey Consortium for Respiratory
    Therapy Education
Saint Clare's Hospital
Dover, NJ

Laura M. Amon, MS, PA-C
Assistant Professor
Physician Assistant Program
Nova Southeastern University
Ft. Lauderdale, FL

Beth Ann Lombardi, B.A.
President and Founder of Impact Communications, Inc.
Johnstown, PA
Senior Technical Writer, Concurrent Technologies Corporation
Johnstown, PA

Joan E. Thiele, PhD, RN
Professor Emeritus
College of Nursing
Intercollege College of Nursing
Washington State University
Spokane, WA

ABOUT THE AUTHOR

Sandra Gaviola, RRT, is a graduate of the University of Pittsburgh at Johnstown. She served as clinical coordinator of The Greater Johnstown Career and Technology Center Respiratory Care Technician Program from 1989 to 1998. She is currently working as a respiratory care practitioner in underserved hospitals throughout the state of Pennsylvania.

While serving as clinical coordinator, the author realized that a majority of students needed help in their student role. The lessons in *My Pocket Mentor* were prepared to help the reader appreciate and enjoy all school-related experiences, setting and attaining goals while accepting the fact that we are only human.

Chapter

1

A PERSONAL AND PROFESSIONAL TRANSFORMATION

Sandra Gaviola

STARTING OVER
  An Opportunity for Personal Growth
  Am I Prepared?

MOTIVATION
  Motivational Behavior
  Rewards
  Overcoming Obstacles

IN THE BEGINNING

LEARNING HABITS
  Making Associations
  Reading
  Listening
  Taking Notes
  Learning to Focus
  Remembering

YOUR REPUTATION
  Honesty
  Determination and Hard Work

So, you are preparing for a career in health care. This time it *really* matters and you are going to . . . do what? Think about that question for a moment—really think about it. Do you see yourself succeeding? Are you excited about the prospects? Are you confident that you have what it takes? Do you *know* what it takes? These are some very important questions to ask yourself. If you answered *no* to any of them, don't worry.

Clearly, success is a process and confidence emerges in time. You are following many former students who answered these same questions with some hesitation. That phase of their career is behind them now as they work in your community and around the world as competent, problem-solving, and caring professionals.

STARTING OVER

Today, many students enrolled in nursing and other allied health care programs know very little about what lies ahead. The most important thing to do is to take only one day at a time, especially in the beginning. Too often, programs experience high attrition (dropout) rates even before the first exam is given. If this sounds familiar, stop and think. Allow yourself some time to adjust to the rigorous workload that comes with higher education. Making the transition from high school or having been out of the classroom for some time will require creative time management as well as lifestyle changes. But what might appear to be an insurmountable feat for you now will slowly evolve into a new routine filled with both sacrifices and rewards. You will find yourself making sacrifices as you develop a mature approach to higher education. And when you are inspired to learn, academic success *is* a realistic goal. Isn't this simple? Having a deeply inspired approach to education results in academic success.

Are you deeply inspired to learn *or* do you want to just get on with it, get that certificate or degree, and begin earning lots of money? Understandably, earning a satisfying income can be a motivational factor, but remember that you won't receive your first paycheck in the near future. Let's begin by exploring other motivational factors that will help you stay on course during the challenging months or years ahead.

An Opportunity for Personal Growth

Your first assignment is this: assess your level of interest in your chosen field of study. Simply ask yourself these questions: *Why am I here? Why did I choose radiology technology, surgical technology, occupational therapy, or dental hygiene as a profession? Who inspired me? What inspired me? What do I know about health care, my earning potential, or shift work?*

PROFESSIONAL GROWTH TIP

The need to have work we love grows as we become older. Not having it can result in paralysis of the spirit.—Author unknown

---

Regardless of the specialty you've chosen or your financial goals, you are likely exceptionally interested in the natural sciences, the human body, and its complex functions. You will learn more about muscles, teeth, red blood cells, adrenaline, the brain, and DNA than you ever thought was possible. You will learn how to handle surgical instruments properly, dress a wound, obtain a history and conduct a physical, floss, passively exercise a trauma patient, reteach a 71-year-old stroke victim how to talk, develop an X-ray, or deliver a baby.

And while all of this is going on, you and your peers will subtly transform on another level: a professional level. *My Pocket Mentor* offers some invaluable lessons that will enable you to grow professionally as you move forward academically. It is highly likely that you will become a "new and improved" individual. Our objective is to provide a unique program that promotes the following qualities:

- Self-awareness
- Effective communication skills
- Professionalism
- Maintenance of physical and emotional health
- Smart money management

By the completion of your formal studies, you will have undergone a rather broad makeover, both academically and personally.

Before we get started, do you have a personal organizer? With every assignment (e.g., technical paper, case study, or worksheet), you are accepting an unspoken agreement that the work will be completed on or before its deadline. A personal organizer will help you to maintain flow and reduce work-related anxiety when you take on each assignment with a specific plan.

Some individuals actually work best under pressure—as the deadline approaches. If working too close to the deadline seems flustering to you, develop the following habits:

- Pace yourself.
- Manage your time.
- Set measurable goals.
- Follow your plan as if it were an exact science.

PROFESSIONAL GROWTH TIP

> *When planning, don't forget to build in some time for playing and resting.*
> *Being a student can be an enjoyable experience despite the workload.*

Am I Prepared?

I entered college for the first time at the nontraditional age of 25. I was not prepared. I graduated from high school with the slightest recollections of chemistry class. My first three-hour college chemistry class was one that I will always remember. The periodic table might as well have been in Greek (although I now know that the symbols are of Latin origin). I was impressed by the ease with which the professor used the periodic table but bothered by the fact that the lecture appeared to be nothing more than a routine chemistry review for most students seated in the classroom. My thoughts during those agonizing three hours? If most of these students have learned this information, then so will I. As my head pounded with all the information that was not adding up very well, I became even more determined. While desperately trying to grasp the information, I was planning the next day. My plan was to rise early and teach myself the value of the periodic table.

Knowing that some students start out at such a disadvantage, you might question what motivates one to stay in the program. Looking back, I realize that it can be somewhat of an evolutionary or developing process.

At the start, I enrolled in an organic chemistry class since it was a basic requirement for most health care professions. The job market was wide open for graduates of health care programs. There was one problem: payday was at least two years away and a steady income was a very distant reward. Interestingly, I felt my incentive to stay engaged in the science of chemistry gradually shifting. I was less focused on a future income and more interested in my classroom performance. I had two weeks before the first exam was to be given and I was neither dropping the class nor failing. In fact, I was determined to do as well or better than the average student. There was no doubt in my mind that I had to work very hard to compete with my classmates. Now I was motivated by the need to succeed.

- I read and reread the chapters.
- I jotted notes frequently.
- I recited formulas out loud when studying.
- I anticipated items that would probably appear on the exam.
- With the textbook closed, I summarized pertinent concepts.

It was paying off and I was grasping the concepts with less effort as we approached midterm.

When the final grades were posted, I saw only two A's and two B's. I'll never know if I finished third or fourth in a class of over 50 students, but I had a feeling of pride knowing that my grade reflected more than my class standing. It reflected my ability to stay motivated despite my lack of a background in chemistry. By this time I was genuinely enjoying the science of chemistry. And now I was motivated by the desire to learn more about health-related sciences.

PROFESSIONAL GROWTH TIP

Expect your motivational factors to evolve along with your appreciation for education.

MOTIVATION

Take a moment to identify the precise event that influenced your decision to enroll in a health care program. Was it your high school guidance counselor's idea? Did your employer permanently lay off workers? Did you realize you needed a higher-paying job? Or did you believe that health care would be an interesting and stimulating profession? Ideally, it was your idea and your curiosity about the field that influenced your decision. You are more likely to stay motivated when you have a real interest in the subject matter.

Motivational Behavior

Motivation is a powerful tool. It can and must be identified and used as a means of achieving your ultimate goals. Motivation is either *intrinsic* (internal) or *extrinsic* (external). Intrinsic motivational behavior is considered more desirable than external motivational behavior, primarily because internal reinforcement is always available. In other words, intrinsic motivation comes from within. It is about the following needs:

- The need to feel informed
- The need to challenge yourself
- The need to satisfy your curiosity about the world around you

Do you see how these concepts are constant and internal and in some ways reflect your values?

Extrinsic motivational behavior can be described as the need to appear intelligent, thereby protecting your ego; the need to make the grade in order to graduate; the pressure to be something that someone else has determined for you or the desire to be rewarded. Despite the negative implications, extrinsic factors can be instrumental in reaching your goals. However, if you function on extrinsic motivational factors alone (salary, for example), you are less likely to achieve real satisfaction at school as well as at work. It's simple: if you're not passionate or enjoying your work, you may begin to experience a number of negative emotions despite a satisfying income.

- Anxiety
- Apathy
- Resentfulness
- A sense of being burdened

PROFESSIONAL GROWTH TIP

> *The most reliable motivational factors are the ones that come from within,*
> *such as your curiosity about the subject matter and your passion to learn.*

Rewards

Recently, I watched an artist whittling human figurines. She was among other fantastic artists showcasing their talents. One piece was positioned especially close to her. She explained to me that this particular piece was a graduation gift she'd whittled for her daughter. The wooden carving was that of an older man seated with his elbows supported on his knees as he narrates *The Princess Diaries*. This work of art was absolutely beautiful. I was impressed by the detail and the artist's ability to capture his pose. I asked her, as she whittled, if she had ever attempted facial detail. *Oh my!* she laughed. *I'm not that talented.* Apparently embarrassed by my next comment, my small group of friends left me standing there alone. My comment to the artist was this: "With little effort, you could capture more detail." I tried to explain to my friends later that this was a compliment. I acknowledged the fact that she already had the *ability*. Given a *motive* (let's say a $5,000 commission), she would have likely made the *effort* to achieve finer detail. It is highly probable that she would put forth the necessary effort, whittling her finest work of all time. Let's apply this to your current role as a student.

- Pre-entrance exams prove that you have the aptitude or *ability*.
- Your desire to learn or need to earn is your *motive*.
- Your *effort* is directly related to your desire to learn or your need to earn.

PROFESSIONAL GROWTH TIP

> *Stay focused on your "commission"—your reward.*

Overcoming Obstacles

A realistic fact of life is that you will be facing obstacles on a regular basis. Some may be minor setbacks while others may require a more involved solution process. Either way, expect setbacks and realize that the sooner you face the challenge and implement a plan of action the sooner you can resume your routine. Always seek professional help when your obstacles are more than you can handle alone or even with a nonprofessional support person.

IN THE BEGINNING

You are only beginning. If you are experiencing some confusion and frustration or feel overwhelmed in the classroom, there is still hope. You have a long way to go. Every day and every event is a learning experience. You can expect some lack of clarity in the beginning. This is normal. But learn as much as you can as soon as you can by staying focused, seeking resources beyond the classroom, searching the Internet for interactive learning tools, and seeking help from individuals who have experience in the field.

You may be weighed down by instructors, guest lecturers, or college professors who are experts in their field and want to convey a heap of information in a short period of time. If the group (in general) agrees that the instructor is moving too quickly and ineffectively, your class representative or a small group can bring this problem to the educator's attention. If your classmates do not share your frustrations, you will have to address this concern on your own. Let your instructor know as early as possible that you are finding it difficult to keep up with the class. Your instructor might suggest hiring a tutor or using other methods of learning until you are acclimated. Prepare yourself for hard work until you have made the adjustment.

———

LEARNING HABITS

In the past 20 years, scientists have actually broadened the definition of intelligence. Educators now believe that true intelligence cannot be measured simply by a test score. It is defined as how well one performs in life. So, if you are questioning whether you are academically prepared to attend a hospital-based or college-level program, consider this: many scientists say that intelligence is only 50 percent inherited; the other half is determined by our life experiences, discipline, and environment. Also, studies show that it is never too late to learn. Maybe now, you can relax and prepare to learn (Michaud & Wild, 1991).

If you think of yourself as an average reader, don't lose sleep. With numerous reading assignments, your ability to comprehend will improve. Continue reading only after you completely comprehend the material already presented. Keep a dictionary on hand. Research the origins of each new word. By doing this, you will steadily broaden your vocabulary. As your vocabulary increases, so will your level of intelligence.

Once you've completed the reading assignment, close the book and from memory write a summary of what you've read. Be sure that you have grasped the general concepts. Then prepare an exam for yourself. With a little luck, you might find some of the same questions on the instructor's exam.

Making Associations

Look for associations with information you have already learned in other classes as the lessons interrelate within the program. Be sure to jot down the associations when you learn them. Writing and visualizing will enable you to retain more information.

Can you make some association or connection in the following example? In medical terminology class you are learning commonly used abbreviations such as BID (twice a day) and TID (three times a day). Knowing that you are in nursing school, your neighbor tells you that his asthma is under control now that he is taking AeroBid. This is a brand-name, long-lasting, anti-inflammatory drug that is taken . . . *How many times a day?* BID is the correct answer.

Try this association. In physics class you will use the delta symbol to indicate change or show a difference. This symbol is shaped like a triangle. The muscle on the upper, outer arm is also shaped like a triangle and is named the deltoid (the suffix *-oid* means "like"). And what about that airline company? The red, white, and blue triangle is Delta's logo resembling the swept wing appearance of a jet. You get the point!

Making associations occurs more frequently as you acquire more knowledge. This means that the more you learn, the more you learn. That was not a typo, that was an association.

Reading

You wouldn't log on to the Internet or leaf through a stack of credit card statements not knowing precisely (or even generally) what you are looking for, would you? Likewise, when you begin a new lesson, find out what you can expect to learn. This can be accomplished in several ways. Start by asking the instructor, *What is the basic premise of this reading assignment?* or, *Precisely what am I expected to learn?* Ask yourself, *Will I discover two separate and completely opposite divisions of the nervous system?* Or, *Will I be focusing on the contrasts and comparisons of sibling rivalry?* Often the author provides the learning objectives before each new section within the text. Too often, they can be overlooked or underused. Still, your instructor is probably your best source for identifying the concepts that must be fundamentally understood.

Listening

Listening is not the same as hearing. *Webster's Dictionary* defines the word *hear* as "to experience or be aware of sounds." The word *listening* is defined as "paying attention to speech." There are a number of reasons we hear but fail to listen. You can name them as well as I can. We've all gotten sidetracked during a lecture. If we have a lack of interest or are preoccupied, we have to work harder at staying focused. Sometimes that's difficult, but you can improve your listening skills by developing the following habits:

- Lean forward and listen intently to concepts under discussion.
- Interact by asking questions at the first appropriate opportunity.
- Avoid taking notes verbatim.
- Avoid mindless highlighting of text.
- In your own words, write a summary of the lecture.
- Draw conclusions.
- Confirm your conclusions with your instructor.
- Enjoy the academic growth spurt. You're growing every day.

Taking Notes

There's an abundance of information regarding note taking. Universities routinely offer note-taking tips to first-year students. This information is also accessible on the Internet. If you feel that you are in need of some direction, check with your school's educational support team or visit other university Web sites.

As your listening skills improve, you will find that your ability to take good notes will as well. I will recommend only one notation style: the one that works for you. Over the years I have seen organized and legible notes (practically a duplicate of the text itself) and I have seen disorganized and illegible notes. As you might guess, the most organized notes are not necessarily written by those who are at the head of the class. Just use the style that works for you. Get creative. Use your own abbreviations or symbols. This is a great time saver. Write vital statements more than once and then underline them. Listen to the speaker's message and focus on the terms or concepts that are reinforced or repeated. Your instructor may be indicating any or all the following:

- This material will be on the exam.
- This concept must be understood in order to learn something more comprehensive.
- This concept must be understood if you are to be a safe practitioner.

By all means, avoid rote learning. This is the practice of learning by memorizing without intelligent understanding. Human physiology and your role in health care must not be reduced to the simple memorization of lists. Ponder the significance of newly presented information and raise the question, *How does this apply clinically?* In other words, what is the usefulness of this information? Develop an inquiring mind. Don't stop at answering the questions. Question the answers.

PROFESSIONAL GROWTH TIP

It's not just your grades that matter. It's what you are learning and what you are doing with the information that matters.

Learning to Focus

MAY I HAVE YOUR ATTENTION?

Concentrate on the content about to be presented. You will be tested on your ability to focus at the end of this session.

The ability to concentrate is an ongoing challenge for students of all ages and academic standings. Lack of concentration is usually the result of one or more of the following:

- Daydreaming
- Anxiety from procrastination
- Unrealistic expectations of being able to study for several hours

Difficulty concentrating can cause feelings of frustration and anxiety that further interfere with your ability to concentrate. Inability to concentrate usually indicates that there is some conflict between studying and other interests that are usually more important to you at the moment than learning. If the inability to focus becomes a problem, you should identify the conflict and then find a solution. Issues involving personal matters can interfere with your need to study. Don't put off addressing these problems. Your school counselor should be available to help. If you find your mind drifting after one hour of reading, take a short break. Do something physical or take a power nap, then return to your books.

Understanding the value of an assignment and how it is to be done will also improve your ability to focus. Communicate with your instructor so that you can establish some learning goals and better direct your thinking. You should have a feeling of satisfaction, not frustration, while studying. Here are some tips to enhance your study habits.

- Managing your time avoids procrastination-related anxiety.
- Clarifying assignments eliminates confusion and frustration.
- Staying engaged in subject matter prevents daydreaming.

Imagine having your first student evaluation. Your instructor hands you a paper filled with various comments on your academic and clinical performance. You are given 10 minutes alone in an office to review the notes. How difficult would it be to focus on this *attention-getter?* You probably wouldn't hear the traffic outside or even the sound of your feet tapping against the legs of the chair. That's concentration.

How was it possible for you to be so focused that you completely blocked out all the sights and sounds around you? Perhaps you were interested in the subject matter (that would be *you*); maybe you were more than just a little curious to learn where you stood; and hopefully you were looking for suggestions on how to reach your peak performance.

What if you could reach the same level of concentration during a 50-minute anatomy and physiology lecture? You can, because you are largely in control of your learning habits. Ask yourself the following questions:

- What's concentration?
- What contributes to concentration?
- What interferes with concentration?
- What will motivate me to change my concentration habits?

At any given moment there are many distractions competing for your attention. It takes conscious effort on your part to focus your attention on what you need to remember. Realize the importance of focusing your attention (this is concentration). In the future, when your mind wanders, make a deliberate attempt to listen more carefully and redirect your attention.

Now close your book and, from memory, answer the following questions: (1) What factors contribute to lack of concentration? (2) What factors interfere with your ability to concentrate? (3) What will you do in the future when your mind starts to wander?

PROFESSIONAL GROWTH TIP

Your efforts to stay focused during a classroom lecture can reduce studying time outside the classroom.

PROFESSIONAL GROWTH TIP

Studying near something that makes a whooshing sound, like a water cooler or a water fountain, can improve concentration by blocking out random, distracting noises (Spiker, 2003).

Remembering

The term *encoding* is used to describe the "process of getting information into long-term memory" (Fogler & Stern, 2001, p. 5). Retaining information in long-term memory can be accomplished by practicing a number of mental tasks. The purpose of practicing these tasks is to give the incoming information more meaning. Try these general tasks for improving your long-term memory:

- Paying attention
- Reasoning it through
- Associating it with something you already know
- Analyzing it
- Elaborating on the details

YOUR REPUTATION

Don't underestimate the consequences of passing off another student's work as your own. This is a delicate issue that instructors face on a regular basis. Cheating (and copying work is cheating), while difficult for instructors to prove, can be grounds for dismissal from the program. Don't put yourself or another member of the class in a position that reflects poorly on those involved. If you go to class with unfinished work, hand it in as is and face the consequences honestly. Your reputation for honesty is more important than turning in work that is doubtfully yours.

Honesty

Yes, it's still the best policy. Honesty is probably the most fundamental quality an individual can possess. You can be described by others in many flattering ways. You may have a positive attitude, great organizational skills, and a sense of humor. But you can't be completely successful unless everything you do is done honestly and with integrity.

PROFESSIONAL GROWTH TIP

You must make a concerted effort to be honorable in all things that you do— at school, at work, and in your social life.

Patients need to feel safe while in your care. They are entitled to the care that is ordered to the letter. For instance, a daily dressing change must be changed daily, a 10-minute passive exercise session must last 10 minutes, and a position change every two hours for a bedridden individual must be done every two hours. In the professional arena, you will be reminded that *if it wasn't charted, it wasn't done.* Electronic and handwritten documentation is essential. There is an even more important reminder: *if it wasn't done, it shouldn't be charted that it was.* Health care professionals are tired of just making do and often fall behind in their workload. It's not uncommon for procedures, therapies, and services in general to be cut short or not be given at all. If a procedure is not done or the therapy time must be reduced due to a staffing shortage, report this to your supervisor or instructor and document the actual length of time or the reason that the services could not be provided. You cannot be held accountable for a staffing shortage; however, you and your institution *can* be held accountable for insurance fraud if the institution is billing for procedures or therapies that were only partially completed or never done.

PROFESSIONAL GROWTH TIP

Don't forget, your reputation is always at stake. So always take the high road with no exceptions.

Determination and Hard Work

Accepting a challenge requires a certain amount of discipline. Of course, there is always the risk of failing. But accepting a challenge is an opportunity to learn more about yourself as you reach higher goals. Determination means looking ahead and expecting to finish, no matter how difficult the task may be.

PROFESSIONAL GROWTH TIP

Regardless of the final outcome, no amount of hard work is ever done in vain.

PERFORMANCE

Your "hands-on" (or psychomotor) skills will improve with practice. Using technical equipment on real patients requires knowledge and skill. Pay special attention to the indications, hazards, and contraindications presented as you learn each new procedure.

Practice, Practice, Practice!

So, how do you reach that higher level of performance? Practice, practice, practice! And when will you feel prepared enough to take your skills to the real world? This will vary among students. It is better to concentrate on the task at hand rather than demand high expectations (of performance) from yourself. Take your time learning each new skill and practice until you feel confident to operate and troubleshoot the specialized instruments and equipment.

Lab Time

Wasting lab time is one of the biggest mistakes a student can make. Lab time is normally built into your schedule. Use it wisely. This is not the time to discuss an upcoming exam with the instructor, copy missed notes, or socialize. You can be the safest and most prepared student only when you use your scheduled lab time wisely. For example, offering to set up the lab is an excellent way to become familiar with the equipment.

A Safe Environment

Students often experience some performance anxiety with each new procedure. Remember, you are not the only one who is experiencing some anxiety and that this is a normal response. Most musicians would probably agree that their best practice sessions are done either alone or in the company of those with whom they feel safe. Discover *your* safe environment and request additional lab time when you and a classmate can run through the procedures at your own pace. Helping another student is a smart way to improve your performance and build your confidence.

I'M ON MY WAY

If you're reading this, you are still with the program and are ready to move along. You probably still have questions about what lies ahead. Again, take one day at a time. Consider this book your personal mentor. It was prepared with your early needs in mind. Together, the authors have logged many student-related experiences, ones that we would like to help you avoid and ones that we would like to see you duplicate.

Making Mistakes

Expect success. But don't expect the school year(s) to be flawless. Learning means making some mistakes. If you don't make some mistakes, you are probably not trying new things. Learn from your slip-ups but don't dwell on them. Jot down the incident if a detailed explanation will prevent you from making the same mistake again. Sharing your learning experiences with your peers can improve the quality of patient care. Finally, be open to constructive criticism. Accept it with appreciation and maturity. Thank the individual who wants to see you succeed.

Raising the Bar

No one ever gets ahead socially or professionally by doing the same things day after day. Times change and we have to make every effort to keep up. I was very inspired not long ago at the U.S. Post Office. Behind the counter was an older man (postretirement age) hammering away on the keys of his computer. He was sharp, he was energetic, and he was up to speed. He was focused and kept the line of customers moving. I was reminded, while observing this older man, how important it is that we never stop raising the bar. Keeping up with technology reflects an individual's progress and helps one maintain skills to perform in "today's" world tomorrow.

Look How Far I've Come

So you've been back in the classroom for how long? You might think it's too early to say, *Look how far I've come.* But it's never too early to utter those words. I encourage you look back occasionally. Ask yourself, *What do I know today that I didn't know at the beginning of this school year?* Looking back, even a short distance, should be enough to encourage you to move forward.

———

A CLASSROOM CONDUCIVE TO LEARNING

Are you familiar with Abraham Maslow's *hierarchy of motives?* According to Maslow (1954, 1971), "our basic needs must be satisfied before our higher needs can be. Maslow's hierarchy of motives states that individuals' main needs are satisfied in the following sequence: physiological, safety, love, belongingness, esteem, and self actualization." For example, you are more likely to satisfy your needs for food before you are motivated to achieve (Santrock, 2000, p. 371).

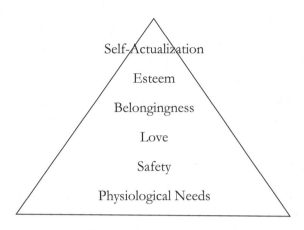

Physical Requirements

While this might seem like a stretch, it's really not. If your physiological needs (e.g., hunger, environmental temperature, or relief from pain) are not met, your ability to move upward on the pyramid to more enjoyable or fulfilling elements is impossible. How can you concentrate on learning if you haven't eaten breakfast, if you are cold, or if you are experiencing the discomfort of a tension headache?

Expect the Unexpected

Take Maslow's advice and come to class prepared. Bring along outerwear, a healthful snack, and something to treat a potential headache. Finally, communicate to your instructor any circumstances that might adversely affect your performance.

HANDLING THE WORKLOAD

Each student will have unique challenges when she or he returns to school. But you will adjust. Don't expect the adjustment to happen immediately. And if your workload and your personal life leave you feeling weary and overwhelmed, keep in mind that it is only temporary. Be specific when communicating your needs to roommates or members of your family. Pace yourself and set aside some time to continue doing the things you enjoy. There is no need to put your entire life on hold. As soon as you adjust to your new routine, you can resume a somewhat normal life.

Solicit the Experienced

Don't miss an opportunity to learn from experienced professionals. Contrary to what we've been told, there really are "dumb questions." So be thoughtful when asking. If you ask an intelligent question, you are more likely to get a comprehensive explanation, as your mentor will sense your level of preparation and interest in your field. Timing is everything. Again, patient safety and care come first. So save your questions for the most appropriate time. You may feel more comfortable when prefacing your questions with, *Do you have a minute? I have a question.* Most individuals are more than willing to answer your questions. Be as brief as possible and thankful for the information.

Here is a list of individuals to whom you may want to address your questions if you haven't reached a sufficient level of comprehension in the subject matter.

- High school teachers
- Professionals who are your personal friends
- Experts who offer interactive services on the Internet
- Tutors for hire

So, you've taken the first serious step by making a commitment to a career in health care. Take your time while reading *My Pocket Mentor.* Remember that this is not only an academic growth spurt but an opportunity for personal and professional development. As you begin your new career, take a look back occasionally. Remember the point at which you started and never lose sight of the professional that you want to become.

REFERENCES

Fogler, J., & Stern, L. (2001). *Improving your memory: How to remember what you're starting to forget.* New York: Barnes & Nobel.

Michaud, E., & Wild, R. (1991). *Boost your brain power.* New York: MJF Books.

Santrock, J. (2002). *Psychology* (6th ed.). New York: McGraw-Hill.

Spiker, T. (2003). Think fast! *Men's Health,* 136–138.

2

AN INSTRUCTOR'S
GOOD ADVICE

Joan E. Thiele

TODAY'S STUDENT

TALKING WITH THE INSTRUCTOR
    Classroom Interaction
    Student-Teacher Interaction
    One-on-One Interaction

SEEKING ASSISTANCE FROM
THE INSTRUCTOR

NEGOTIATING

STUDENT RESPONSIBILITY
AND ACCOUNTABILITY
    Active Participation
    Active Learning
    Understanding the Assignment

INSTRUCTOR RESPONSIBILITY
AND ACCOUNTABILITY
Logical Sequence Presentation
Fair and Impartial Performance Evaluation

PERSONALITY CONFLICTS
    Differences in Perception
    What to Do?

STUDENT-INSTRUCTOR CULTURAL
DIFFERENCES

UNDESIRABLE CLASSROOM
BEHAVIOR
    Technology in the Classroom
    Disruptive Activity
    Special Concessions and
        Thoughtless Questions
    Verbal Misconduct

THE CLINICAL ENVIRONMENT
    Professional Behavior
    Performance Standards
    Learning From Clinical Experience
    Patient Care Considerations
    Clinical Evaluation

Whether you've just graduated from high school or have been in the workforce for several years, moving on to higher education can be a scary proposition. Individuals who go straight to college from high school must adapt to being away from home and learn to balance their academic requirements with their personal lives. For these students, adjusting to college includes meeting new friends, planning schedules, and fulfilling the requirements of multiple courses. For nontraditional students, their lives will change in a different way, as they will have to keep up their usual household responsibilities while meeting the challenges that higher education has to offer.

TODAY'S STUDENT

Today, only one-third of university students are ages 18 to 24 (Risser, 2002). The remaining two-thirds of the college population are between the ages of 25 and 44. The nontraditional student is typically a parent, working part-time and attending school (Medved & Heisler, 2002). The multiple roles managed by students consume a tremendous amount of time and energy and can pose a challenge to both the instructor and the student.

PROFESSIONAL GROWTH TIP

Asking questions directly related to the concepts presented in class will help you understand the course content. This one action, asking questions, contributes most to success in college.

TALKING WITH THE INSTRUCTOR

To a busy student, taking the time to talk with an instructor may seem to be an unnecessary activity. Remember, instructors are in the business of higher education. Their success is measured by student success. Talking with the instructor, particularly in relation to course activities, is one action that significantly improves student motivation, attitude toward school, and success in a program (Medved & Heisler, 2002). However, simply approaching the instructor and saying, *Hey, we need to talk!* is not going to have positive outcomes. Give a specific purpose for wanting to meet with your instructor while acknowledging that professors and instructors have posted office hours.

Classroom Interaction

Often, a student raises thought-provoking questions that challenge other learners to explore the relevance of the content being taught to real-life events. However, students in a large lecture classroom of 100 to 200 learners may allow their questions to go unspoken because they are reluctant to question the instructor during or after class. Students who frequently ask questions of the instructor during class are more likely to succeed in college and to complete their degrees than are the silent individuals.

Student-Teacher Interaction

The vast majority of student-teacher interactions relate to the course. Since the class in which both student and instructor are participating is one element that both parties have in common, discussing course-related topics is a natural occurrence. These discussions also provide students with an excellent opportunity to ask those unspoken questions. Often, students do not understand the course material completely or question how the information is to be used. The instructor is the most appropriate individual to ask for additional clarification. Asking your classmates to clarify content may add to your confusion. They, too, may not have understood some of the concepts. For clarification of lecture content, approaching the instructor immediately after class with a brief question is most appropriate. Asking for additional clarification immediately after a lecture on a topic will help you learn the material and retain it correctly for future use, such as for the next examination.

PROFESSIONAL GROWTH TIP

Asking content-related questions is an indication of interest in the course on your part and helps to establish and to maintain a positive student-teacher relationship.

One-on-One Interaction

Questions that require more than a few minutes to answer or those from content from several classes ago are best answered in the instructor's office. Simply ask your instructor when you may meet to discuss some of the course material. In this way, the instructor is able to select a time when you will be given full attention and you are not in a position to delay the instructor from getting to the next class or a faculty meeting. Writing your questions in advance will help you organize your thinking and identify the material that you need to have clarified. A written list also means that you will be prepared to take notes on the answers as you and the instructor discuss the material. Be specific with your questions. For example, say, *I don't understand the relationship between A and B,* rather than, *Tell me all I need to know about A and B.* In order to use your time and that of the instructor most effectively, you need to review your notes and the information in the textbook prior to meeting with the instructor. I found that an effective process for me was to rewrite my notes and fill in the blank areas and missing content from the textbook. As I did this, I wrote my questions in the margins next to the incomplete or misunderstood content. With my notes as a guide, I could quickly locate my questions and jot down the answers that the instructor provided. To me, this process was an efficient use of everyone's time. My complete notes were much better for study purposes than were the sketchy and incomplete jottings recorded during class. You will find a note-taking style that works best for you.

Other topics that are best discussed in the instructor's office are specific test questions and/or test results. While it is tempting to do this in the classroom, unless the instructor offers to review a test with the total class, your questions may not be of interest to your classmates. Rather than force them to waste time on items that are not of their concern, approach the instructor after class and arrange a meeting time in the privacy of the individual's office. In this way, you receive information pertaining to the answers you selected on the test. The instructor can clarify any misunderstandings you have regarding the content and offer suggestions that may assist you on future tests. Arguing with the instructor regarding particular test items and their intended answers is usually a fruitless activity. Rather, when you meet with the instructor to discuss your test, bring your source(s) of information with you. In this way, you provide the rationale for the answer you selected. Do not be surprised, however, if your instructor does not allow you to spend a great deal of time perusing your individual responses to various items. Rather, he or she will likely encourage you to learn to make content connections and to think critically about application of the content. As a student entering a health science profession it is imperative for you to develop the ability to determine content application in multiple situations rather than simply memorizing responses to fact-specific questions. In other words, analyze rather than memorize.

Often, misperceptions of information by the student, the teacher, or both, are identified. Teachers write questions based upon their knowledge of a subject. However, students often interpret questions in a manner that is different from the intent of the item writer. Reviewing test items with an instructor reveals these different interpretations. Once the problem is identified, a solution is easy to determine. This approach demonstrates respect for both the student's and the instructor's points of view.

PROFESSIONAL GROWTH TIP

The focus of such discussions (regarding different interpretations) is on learning, not on who is right or wrong.

SEEKING ASSISTANCE FROM THE INSTRUCTOR

Instructors are in a unique position to provide information to students in relation to a multitude of campus services. Meeting with an instructor or an advisor is a smart way to identify sources of support that may contribute to academic and personal success. Services often provided by colleges include tutoring, writing, counseling, academic advising, babysitting, health care for you and your children, and financial assistance. These services are designed to assist students in achieving success in their academic pursuits. Use of these services is a benefit to all college students. These services are usually built into the cost of your education, so take advantage of their availability.

NEGOTIATING

At some point, you may need to negotiate with an instructor in relation to an individual request. The request may be an extension of a due date for a paper, making up a missed examination, or completion of an assignment that was not submitted. Remember that instructors are human; they, too, have sick children, become ill themselves, and engage in multiple time-consuming activities outside of the classroom. Arrange to meet with your instructor, and then briefly explain the extenuating circumstances. Generally, a factual statement of reality, *My child was sick,* or, *I had a flat tire on my way to class* is the preferred approach for making a request, rather than an emotional appeal based on values, a sense of fairness, or other individual principles. Offer a specific plan for completing the assignment, paper, or other activity. Then, allow the instructor to present a counter-offer. The instructor may suggest other options that you had not considered. After reviewing the suggested completion options, both of you need to agree upon a specific date and time that is realistic for completion of the missing work. Be sure to write down the terms of the agreement. Your instructor will also make a note of the agreement and hold you responsible for meeting the specified terms. Once the request is granted, fulfilling the commitment is your responsibility. Be careful, however, that you do not ask for extended time for every paper and examination. Such behavior is indicative of procrastination and poor time management rather than being a single unavoidable event that interrupted your time schedule.

PROFESSIONAL GROWTH TIP

The art of negotiating requires that each side give a little.

STUDENT RESPONSIBILITY AND ACCOUNTABILITY

Responsibility and accountability are thrust upon students. You are responsible for getting to class or obtaining information should you miss a class. Your classmates are not the best source of information about class content. Remember that in the typical class, a student writes down only a small percentage of what was actually said. These written words may be disjointed and miss the critical points entirely. Perhaps the attention of the classmate wandered at some point and an entire section of content was missed. You take responsibility by asking the instructor if there is some way that you can obtain the content you missed. Perhaps the class was videotaped for later transmission; if so, ask for permission to view the tape. On occasion, an instructor will review the notes with you in a private session in her or his office. Or, the instructor may have other suggestions. In any event, simply ignoring the content from the missed class does not exempt you from being held accountable for learning the material. Your responsible actions contribute to your academic success.

Active Participation

Many of your courses may require your active participation. Health care careers require interaction and communication with multiple individuals on a daily basis. The courses that you take provide an opportunity to learn effective communication techniques. Active participation in courses often means more than simply going to the class. You may be asked to interview others, to document your activities, and to practice application of the communication techniques presented in class (Peterson, 2001). Below is a list of other activities in which you may be required to participate in class.

- Speaking before the class
- Responding to questions about the content

- Presenting your interpretation of the information and defending your views

All of these learning activities are designed to help you to think critically about the material, explore its meaning, and use the content in simulated (or imitated) situations.

Active Learning

Active learning demands careful listening to the comments and viewpoints presented by fellow students. Responding to the questions presented by others and analyzing problem situations are a part of active learning. These types of activities prepare you to "think on your feet," or to respond as you will be expected to do when actually providing care to patients. Allow the instructor or professor to respond to questions presented by other students. Interrupting or attempting to "help" when another student poses a question may cause confusion and waste valuable time. Allow the instructor to handle the question alone unless the opportunity to clarify the content is open to the class.

PROFESSIONAL GROWTH TIP

Preparation outside of the classroom is essential for students to be active, participating learners in the classroom.

Budgeting your time to allow for preparation prior to class is essential for health care students. Learning the content is a vital starting point. Active learning helps students to think critically and to practice interpersonal skills of listening, speaking, and communicating effectively with others. For many students, the transition from a traditional lecture-based class to an active learning class is difficult to make. Knowing in advance that participation beyond passive note taking will be demanded of you will make this transition easier. If you are not certain of the expectations of your instructor, be sure to ask for an explanation and examples of the forms of participation to be demonstrated. While the instructor is responsible for providing clear directions and illustrations, you will be expected to demonstrate the following activities to adjunct (additional) faculty outside the classroom.

- Demonstration of your critical thinking
- Understanding of the content and its application
- Effective communication with other professionals

All of these activities are preparation for the challenges you will face in the realities of working in the health care arena.

Understanding the Assignment

Not understanding what the instructor wants in relation to a particular assignment or activity is a reality. The solution is simple: ask the instructor for examples and a better explanation of what the outcome is to be. When creating an assignment, the instructor has an idea as to the final product; however, that idea may not have been fully transmitted to students. The instructor is responsible for creating assignments and making them understandable to the learners in a course. Do not hesitate to go to the instructor when you do not understand the expectations. I know that when I write a set of directions on how to prepare a spreadsheet, I often omit steps just because I know how to do them. However, the novice learner who has never created a spreadsheet cannot automatically insert the missing steps. The same thing happens to other instructors in relation to development of their course assignments. You can be of great assistance to the instructor by pointing out the gaps in the assignment. Ask questions that require clarification of the activity and identify the missing steps.

PROFESSIONAL GROWTH TIP

Your responsibility is to make sure you understand the assignment so that you can perform to your highest level.

PROFESSIONAL GROWTH TIP

You can be of great assistance to the instructor by pointing out the gaps in an assignment.

INSTRUCTOR RESPONSIBILITY AND ACCOUNTABILITY

Just as you have new responsibilities as a student, your instructor also has responsibilities to you and the profession in general. Foremost among these is to teach well. That means that teachers are expected to present lectures that are as clear as possible to foster student understanding. You can expect instructors to use a planned sequence of events in presenting a lecture.

Logical Sequence Presentation

First, the instructor will typically begin with an overview. The opening statements may be something such as, *Today's class is about* . . . Next, the material will be organized so that a step-by-step logical sequence of information emerges. For example, if the topic of discussion is diabetes mellitus, you should expect the instructor to begin with a definition and the pathophysiology of the disease. Following this, the two major classifications are described. Then, symptoms of diabetes exhibited by the individual are portrayed. Lastly, today's treatment methods are examined. As you can see, this sequence of content is designed to build systematically upon your knowledge of the disease.

Following this sequenced presentation, the instructor will provide examples that illustrate the major points and solicit questions from students. This enables students to review their notes and ask for clarification of information that was not clear to them. Remember, asking questions forces you to use the content appropriately and enhances your learning.

PROFESSIONAL GROWTH TIP

The offer by the instructor to answer questions is an opportunity you will want to use frequently.

The remaining step in the instructional sequence is to assess your knowledge of this content. In clinical courses, you will be expected to apply the information accurately as you assess and care for individuals with various forms of diabetes. Lecture courses will use an examination approach to assess your knowledge.

Fair and Impartial Performance Evaluation

Your instructor is also responsible for fair and impartial evaluation of your performance. Evaluation is a daunting task for instructors, as decisions made affect students in a multitude of ways. Every effort is made to perform this task in a conscientious and honest manner. Being human, instructors make mistakes and may inadvertently develop inaccurate evaluations. Mathematical errors, poor record keeping, losing a paper, or simply misinterpreting a student's actions all contribute to incorrect evaluation results. If this happens to you, remember that the academic system offers a multitude of protections for the rights of students. Should you be in the position of receiving a grade that you think is not consistent with your performance, your first recourse is to speak privately with the instructor. Take your records of your performance with you and ask for an explanation of the difference between your calculated grade and that of the instructor. After discussing the issue, most of the grade disputes are resolved. If, however, you are not satisfied with the outcome, your next recourse is to speak with the instructor's immediate supervisor. In most instances, the visit to the instructor's office results in resolution of the dispute.

PROFESSIONAL GROWTH TIP

Your student handbook will provide the chain of command and specific instructions and steps to be taken to resolve grade disputes.

Throughout the grade review process, mutual respect is to be demonstrated. You and the instructor are both responsible for listening to one another's views and respecting your differences. Failure to do so by either you or the instructor is dodging responsibility. Simply deciding that you have a "personality conflict" with the instructor will not resolve the issues at hand. While you may disagree with the instructor's viewpoint, your best action is to listen carefully to the evidence presented by the instructor to support the assigned grade. Following this, offer your view and other information regarding your performance. An effective presentation of your learning and application of the course material often results in a mutually agreed-upon grade that is consistent with your level of performance.

___

PERSONALITY CONFLICTS

What if you have a personality conflict with an instructor? What does this really mean? Keep in mind that you probably do not know your instructor well enough to have more than a superficial knowledge of his or her personality and only that piece displayed in the classroom. More than likely, your instructor did not grow up in an age of intensive technological development. The difference in age accounts for many personality conflicts. Since you cannot age rapidly or make the instructor younger, each of you must respect one another's views. This does not mean that you must agree with the instructor; it simply means that you acknowledge that you each have different views on some subjects and that you accept these differences.

> ## PROFESSIONAL GROWTH TIP
>
> *Often, what is perceived as a "personality conflict" is actually two different perceptions of events. Because of your difference in life experiences or values, your instructor and you may not see the events in the same light.*

Differences in Perception

Student comments such as *My teacher doesn't like me because I am of a different race or religious group,* or, *My teacher wants me to fail this course,* or, *There is a personality conflict between my instructor and me* are indicators of differences in perception. Teachers may have their own biases; however, in this day and age considerable focus has been placed upon the importance of recognizing cultural differences or differences in personal values. Instructors are responsible for accepting individuals of all races and creeds without making judgments based upon these differences. Failure to do so is a very serious charge and may be grounds for dismissal of the instructor. A more appropriate interpretation is that the instructor does not share your view or simply does not understand your perceptions.

What to Do?

In such circumstances, make an appointment to talk with the instructor and share your concerns. An opening statement may be something such as, *It's my feeling that you may dislike me because . . .* In this way, you place the issue on the table and allow both of you to explain your views. Open communication is a sure-fire method of resolving individual issues and clarifying misperceptions.

In all of my years of teaching, I have never known a teacher who wanted a student to fail. The statement, *My instructor wants me to fail,* is simply the student's perception. If a student is failing, it is because of a variety of reasons. The most common reason for failing a course is lack of time and attention to the content. Ask yourself what it is that you are doing to contribute to your success in the classroom. This is *your* responsibility, not the instructor's. You may need to adjust your study schedule to allow sufficient time for you to learn the material presented in class.

PROFESSIONAL GROWTH TIP

Remember that each class requires two to three hours of study time outside of the classroom per hour of course credit.

STUDENT-INSTRUCTOR CULTURAL DIFFERENCES

You and your instructor may be from vastly different cultures, a factor that can contribute to misunderstanding. The instructor may be very naïve about your culture and your expectations of instructors. In such circumstances, you can be of great assistance to the instructor. For example, you may need to (privately) provide the instructor with the correct pronunciation of your name, or the name by which you prefer to be called. Misperceptions are easily corrected by providing accurate information to a willing listener. If you are going to miss class due to a culturally related activity, explain this to the instructor before the event. At the same time, make arrangements for obtaining the class content you will miss.

While instructors are learning to be aware of cultural biases in test questions, these still may be found in their examinations. Discuss the concepts with the instructor and point out the differences in perception of the questions based on your culture. Instructors are not "mind readers"; they cannot know that the words they used have a different interpretation in your culture. For example, one nursing instructor asked a question about nutrition in the older patient; the answer suggested that providing prunes as part of the diet would be beneficial. An Asian student later talked to the instructor and asked, *What are prunes?* The student knew the content but not the context in which the question was presented. Thus, a cultural perception that everyone would understand the question was found to be erroneous. (Yes, the student received credit for the question, as she understood the concept underlying the question.) The instructor changed the question to better address the student's culture.

Individuals from non-Western cultures often find it difficult to understand psychiatric illnesses, as these types of illnesses may not be recognized as such. Other individuals may have difficulty accepting the scientific discipline and research base of Western medicine. These differences are real but need not interfere with one's learning. The instructor is asking that you learn and understand information, not that you subscribe to a particular point of view or philosophy.

UNDESIRABLE CLASSROOM BEHAVIOR

While it seems strange to discuss appropriate classroom behavior at the college level, changes in student attitudes and views of correct behavior make this a necessity. A frequent topic of discussion among college faculty is inappropriate classroom behavior of students. In this age of road rage and multiple other forms of violent behaviors, the classroom has become a place in which new student behaviors are emerging. Not all of these behaviors are acceptable, as they disrupt the learning environment of the classroom. Some of the more common forms of unacceptable behavior are described below. These were obtained by asking instructors to describe the classroom behaviors they found particularly annoying.

Technology in the Classroom

The use of computers, digitized media, and other electronic enhancements for teaching purposes has contributed greatly to the instructor's ability to provide lectures that are clear and supplemented with visual examples. However, use of computers by students during the course of a lecture is not always acceptable. Many instructors deem students' use of computers, especially to play games or send electronic messages, during a lecture unacceptable. Obviously, the students are not attending to the material being presented and may be distracting other students.

Lectures are the primary teaching method for many instructors; inattentive behaviors by students are a major contributor to incorrect interpretations and difficulty passing courses. In fact, one individual stated "teachers in most institutions spend 80 percent of their time lecturing to students, who in turn are attentive some 50 percent of the time" (Butler, as cited in Peterson, 2001). Inattentive behaviors are distracting to other students and contribute to a lack of comprehension of the content of the course.

PROFESSIONAL GROWTH TIP

Before using a computer to record notes, ask your instructor if this is permissible.

Some instructors are in agreement with the use of electronic devices in the classroom, others find it distracting to other individuals in the classroom and do not allow computers to be used during their classes.

One behavior that is unanimously not acceptable to instructors is using a cell phone during class. As cell phones have increased in popularity, so, too, has their use in inappropriate places. Think of yourself as being deeply absorbed in answering a difficult anatomy test question. Suddenly the cell phone of the person sitting next to you rings. There goes your concentration. Of course, the person feels a need to answer the ringing phone. Although a low tone of voice is used, the conversation is audible to individuals in the immediate vicinity. This type of behavior has prompted many college instructors to ban cell phones from the classroom. Certainly, there are times when you must be in a position to be contacted by others. Simply adjust your cell phone to vibrate and step outside the room if you believe a call must be answered immediately.

Disruptive Activity

Noises that disrupt others need to be held to a minimum in class. Another behavior that instructors find disruptive is the loud student who arrives late for class. This individual typically allows the door to bang upon entering the classroom and noisily takes a seat. After ripping the Velcro straps from a backpack to retrieve a notebook and pen, the individual is ready to attend to the lecture. During this process, everyone in the class has had difficulty hearing the instructor and has become very inattentive. Several minutes of precious class time have been lost through this individual's behaviors, the attention of the class has been shattered, and the patience of the instructor has been sorely tried. More important, repeated episodes of this behavior result in a significant reduction in the amount of time available for presentation of content, discussion of examples, and answering of student questions.

If you are late for class, enter the room quietly. Consistent tardiness on your part is also a behavior that instructors find unacceptable. Remember that the overview of the class discussion is presented in the first few minutes. Missing this important information means that you do not have the advanced organizer that will increase your understanding of the content being presented. Your notes may be disorganized due to missing the overview, which outlined what the lecture was about.

Another behavior that is sure to irritate an instructor is students talking to each other while the instructor is lecturing. Many times, such conversations have nothing to do with the instructor's presentation. The noise of the conversation is enough to distract the instructor and other students in the class. The instructor may politely ask the perpetrators about the conversation or if there is some question about the content. Repeated episodes of talking may result in your being asked to leave the classroom.

Special Concessions and Thoughtless Questions

A difficult concept for students to consider is that once class begins, the instructor is in charge—completely. Keep in mind that a classroom is not a democracy. For example, you will not be asked to vote on whether to have a test or when your paper is due. When the course was designed, the instructor made these decisions based upon knowledge of a logical sequence of information and appropriate times or points for changing topics. In addition, the instructor planned content with full knowledge of the academic calendar.

Another unacceptable behavior is the asking of thoughtless questions. Questions such as *Do we have to turn in our papers on Monday?* fit this category. This question is easily answered by thoroughly reading the course syllabus and course calendar. Guidelines for papers and other required activities will be provided. Another example of a thoughtless question is asking the same thing that the instructor just answered. New questions that expand upon the content are always welcome; however, items that are of interest to only you are to be addressed outside of the classroom setting. The instructor is attentive to the time allotted to the class and will attempt to use each minute in a manner that fosters learning by *all* students.

Verbal Misconduct

Verbal abuse and inappropriate language, particularly racial slurs, vulgarity, and profanity, are not tolerated in the classroom. Verbal abuse can take many forms, but is often a statement that is perceived as a threat or challenge by the instructor. As you learn communication techniques, you will become more aware of the types of statements that are considered verbal abuse. Repeated verbal abuse or use of profanity in the classroom may result in your removal from the course. This type of conduct is grounds for dismissal in the workplace.

PROFESSIONAL GROWTH TIP

A learning environment does not have to be silent; busy, engaged, participating students are a delight to the instructor.

PROFESSIONAL GROWTH TIP

When you make a verbal statement, be attentive to the language you use.

THE CLINICAL ENVIRONMENT

By their very nature, health care disciplines incorporate some amount of practice in the actual clinical environment. Caring for patients for the first time often invokes anxiety in students. In the following paragraphs, expectations for students in the clinical arena are explored.

Professional Behavior

Students in a clinical practice setting are held to the same standards of conduct and performance as licensed professionals in the field. Being a student places tremendous responsibility upon you. You must act like your instructors and the other professionals from whom you are learning. Imagine *your* response to the following situation:

You are the parent of a 12-month-old infant who has a high temperature and has been hospitalized to receive intravenous fluids and antibiotics. Soon after admission, a student nurse enters the room. After giggling for a few minutes and commenting, *Oh, what a cute baby!* she tells you that she is going to perform a lung assessment, that is, listen to the breathing of the child (rate, rhythm, and sounds). She fumbles with her stethoscope, listens quickly to the front of the child's chest on the left side, writes notes on a scrap of paper, giggles again, and leaves. If you were the parent of this child, how do you think you would respond?

Obviously, this student had very little knowledge about what she was doing or how to go about a true assessment. As the parent, you could request that students not be allowed to care for your child. In fact, such a request is not unusual. Prove that you are knowledgeable so that all patients and/or their parents and guardians feel safe in your care.

Performance Standards

As a student in a health care profession, your responsibility is to perform to the standards of practicing individuals. This means that you must become competent in the performance of multiple actions. Whether you are learning to be a respiratory therapist, dental hygienist, or registered nurse, practicing skills that you will perform on real patients is mandatory. Many institutions provide simulated (imitation) clinical labs for this very purpose. In the practice lab, you can gain competence and confidence in your ability to use the various instruments and technical equipment required for your discipline. Once you feel competent in the lab, you will advance to clinical sites where real patients will be receiving your care.

Another set of skills that you will practice are those of interviewing and communicating with patients. Giggling your way through an interview or asking irrelevant questions is not the performance you would expect of someone who is caring for your sick child or anyone else. Practice of the required skills in a nonthreatening environment is the way to develop your performance abilities and to avoid acting like the student presented in the above scenario.

Another aspect of clinical performance is your personal appearance. Many of the health-related disciplines will require students to wear a uniform. If the uniform is simply a laboratory coat or jacket, your other attire is considered to be part of your total dress. Adherence to the standards set forth in your student handbook is mandatory. These standards typically address wearing of nail polish, jewelry, and perfumes or aftershave lotion. Health care institutions also may have their set of standards of appearance for employees. As a student, you will be held to the same standards as employees of the institution in which you are a student. Your initial orientation to a new clinical setting will include a review of the appearance students are required to observe. Failure to meet these standards may result in your being dismissed from your program or receiving an unsatisfactory grade in a clinical course.

Learning From Clinical Experience

Being a student in a health discipline is often difficult; expect and accept it. You are expected to perform like a professional, yet you do not have the knowledge or expertise to do so. What are you to do? First of all, acknowledge your limitations. If you have never performed a certain procedure, position yourself to observe it and practice it in the simulated lab before doing so on a hospitalized individual.

Develop the habit of asking questions. Why, how, and when questions will help you expand your understanding of patient care. Don't hesitate to ask your instructors, other professionals, and patients for explanations that will broaden your understanding and increase your confidence.

Patient Care Considerations

The cardinal rule of patient care is, *Do no harm.* As a student, if you do not know how to do something, do not attempt to muddle through a procedure on a patient. Simply telling your supervisor *I don't know* is sufficient. At that point, you will be instructed in the correct procedure and supervised in your performance, or someone with the expertise will perform the required procedure. Your responsibility is to learn the information you need so that you will be able to perform the procedure later. In all events, do no harm.

Clinical Evaluation

Your performance in the clinical arena will be evaluated. In some disciplines, satisfactory clinical performance is as critical, or even more so, than grades on the didactic, or clinical, component of your curriculum. You may be dismissed from a program for unsatisfactory clinical performance. In the event that you disagree with your instructor's evaluation of your performance, you may use this log to compare perceptions of your performance. Be sure that you read the clinical course syllabus; the performance expectations will be outlined in this handout. If you do not understand the performance requirements, be sure to ask the instructor. Factual knowledge is a must, but excellence in clinical performance is a mandate. Learn all you can and develop your performance abilities at every opportunity.

PROFESSIONAL GROWTH TIP

Keep a log or journal of your experiences and learn from the clinical events.

This chapter presented an overview of didactic course and clinical performance expectations of students in various health care professions. Hopefully, these expectations presented from the view of a clinical and didactic instructor will help you understand your role as a health care student. Above all, learn, learn, and learn. And, enjoy the experience!

REFERENCES

Medved, C. M., & Heisler, J. (2002). A negotiated order exploration of critical student-faculty interactions: Student parents manage multiple roles. *Communication Education, 51*(2), 105–120.

Peterson, R. M. (2001). Course participation: An active learning approach employing student documentation. *Journal of Marketing Education, 233,* 187–194.

Risser, P. (2002). Speech cited in Gelhausen, M. Portland keynote address highlighted OSU programs and educational changes that are facing universities. *Cost Engineering, 44*(10), 6–9.

3

WRITE A
TECHNICAL PAPER?
WHEN IS IT DUE?

Beth Ann Lombardi

TURN WORRY INTO WORK
Know Your Audience
Know Your Assignment Parameters
Know Your Style Guide
Know the Different Forms of Writing
Know the Tone of Technical Writing

RESEARCH
Primary Research
Secondary Research

IMMERSE YOURSELF IN THE TOPIC
Writing the Paper in Your Own Words

THINK, THEN TYPE
Motivators
The Craft of the Draft

EDIT!
Steps to Quality Editing
Watch for These Common Mistakes
Repairing Sentences
Proofreader Marks

BYLINES AND BLISTERS

Have you heard of white-coat anxiety? It occurs when a patient's blood pressure increases at the sight of a doctor, a nurse, or any official-looking person in a white lab coat. In this chapter, I'd like to talk about blank-white-paper anxiety—the fear of facing a blank sheet of paper or computer screen in anticipation of writing a technical document.

Even if you dread writing so much that you're considering skipping this chapter, there's help for you. Yes, writing is hard work, but it's hardly boring. It's usually a solo job, most easily accomplished alone, but not necessarily in solitude. Good writing requires self-discipline, a desire to communicate well, and a measure of creativity. Even if you're writing a technical paper, you have to dance with the words, making them work in sync with each other and with your intended message.

Refuse to let that blank white sheet of paper intimidate you. Writing a paper isn't a big deal. Here's my formula: WRITE!

- **W**orry, then **w**ork
- **R**esearch
- **I**mmerse yourself in the topic
- **T**hink, then **t**ype
- **E**dit!

TURN WORRY INTO WORK

Even professional writers experience a degree of fear when beginning a new project. Feel better knowing you're not the only one who's ever had blank-white-paper anxiety? Think I didn't worry when I accepted this assignment? Think I didn't ask myself if I could top my last article, find a new and unique way to communicate well, and deliver ideas that would make a difference in readers' lives?

To turn worry into work, I convert the energy and time I start spending on worrying into the motivation I need to get the project done. Someone once told me that you either worry or you work. That works for me. Let's make it work for you, too.

Begin by collecting essential information about your assignment. Before you write, you need to identify your audience as well as the style guide and any specific parameters that have been established for your paper. We'll discuss these three items just as soon as you digest your first quick tip for writing a technical paper.

PROFESSIONAL GROWTH TIP

Home in on a subject and write a mission statement that clearly defines the objective of your paper.

A 35-year veteran technical writer who reviewed the draft of this chapter for me said he had never been told to write a mission statement. I explained that he may not find the idea in other books but it is an idea that works well for me, and I am confident that others will benefit from its use. The exercise of developing mission statements will extend into other areas of education and business, helping you develop a strategic, logical thought process for all projects.

You'll refer to your mission statement again and again throughout the writing process. Like the North Star, the mission statement is your focal point. Never lose sight of it, and your paper will stay on course.

Sample mission statements:

- This paper will discuss the benefits and drawbacks of a new blood-pressure treatment.
- This paper will discuss recent changes in guidelines for neonatal resuscitation.

Know Your Audience

Who will read and benefit from your effort? Is the intended reader a health care professional? Is the reader likely to understand basic medical jargon such as outpatient (a patient who is not admitted for an overnight stay in a hospital) or CBC (complete blood count)? If the reader might not know that an angiocath is an IV, you have identified one of the most important things you need to keep in mind when writing your paper. Know your reader and use vocabulary familiar to him or her.

Still confused? Consider the difference between the wonderfully creative A. A. Milne's prose in *The Complete Works of Winnie the Pooh* (Dutton, 1994) and best-selling author Danielle Steel's writing style in *Sunset in St. Tropez* (Delacorte Press, 2002). Compare the word choice and sentence structure of an article in the *Journal of American Medicine* with one in *USA Today*. Write for your audience; meet their needs.

Know Your Assignment Parameters

Format—fonts, margins, footnote style, how to handle attribution, and more—can set your paper apart from other submissions. Get answers to housekeeping questions such as these when you are first assigned the paper. How many pages or words are expected? Are there any special restrictions? When is the paper due? Ask which style guide you should use; as you'll read in the following section, it's an important resource.

Know Your Style Guide

A style guide provides writers with the rules of style for a particular document or organization (such as a school, business, or publishing house). It offers guidance on such topics as accepted abbreviations, capitalization, titles, and more. Good style guides establish clear, easy-to-follow rules, ensuring cohesion and readability.

I was once involved with a committee that spent nearly a year assembling a corporate style guide. One of the biggest debates: use of the series comma (for example: "Writing is fun, energizing and rewarding" or "Writing is fun, energizing, and rewarding"). Should the comma precede the conjunction in a simple series? Both sides came out slugging. Tempers flared. Meetings became debates. Writers became warriors. The *Chicago Manual of Style* endorses the series comma; the *Associated Press Stylebook and Libel Manual* does not (except in the instance of a complex series of phrases). Countless other style guides were consulted before putting the issue up for a good ole democratic vote. The group agreed to do away with the comma before the conjunction in the last item of a series. There was a collective sigh of relief that the issue was finally resolved. That is how important a style guide is.

Should you use *healthcare* or *health care*? *On-line* or *online*? *Web site, website,* or *web site*? Ever noticed these minute differences? Technical writers live (and I dare say that many thrive) on these minute differences in the language.

PROFESSIONAL GROWTH TIP

Be consistent. Consistency enhances the readability of documents.

If you write *healthcare* once, use *healthcare* throughout the document, never *health care*. If you're consistent, it's hard for any editor or professor to pull out a red pen. Moreover, if you're consistent, the reader will be more apt to understand your message.

Know the Different Forms of Writing

Technical writing deals with topics relating to the medical, computer, engineering, and science industries. Technical writing is precise and academic in nature.

It may be easier to tell you what technical writing is *not*. It is not advertising, storytelling, fiction, grant writing, journalism, copy writing, editorial writing . . . or anything but technical writing. Technical writers usually communicate highly complex ideas and innovations. Often, the purpose of a technical paper is to introduce or substantiate a new concept or to explain a promising new scientific procedure. Articles are published in industry-specific journals to help advance the field of study. Much hinges on the technical writer's ability to explain difficult or new (or both) ideas clearly and concisely and to avoid any unnecessary clutter that may detract from the message.

I was once asked to write about laparoscopic surgery early in its history. I read articles in medical journals, studied the literature prepared by companies that marketed laparoscopes, and interviewed patients. Doctors invited me into the operating room to observe the new procedure. To make sure I understood how laparoscopic procedures compared with traditional surgery, I also observed an invasive gallbladder operation. The doctor proudly noted as he delved a gloved hand deep into his patient's abdomen, "The laparoscope is okay, but I love getting my hands into the belly. *That's* real surgery." I got the picture and did my best to communicate honestly and clearly the nuances of this cutting-edge technology.

> When describing laparoscopic surgery in an advertisement, copy blazoned: "Cutting-edge surgery without the cut." "You'll enjoy a quicker recovery." "Why have a five-inch scar when you can avoid it?"

> When describing laparoscopic surgery in an editorial, I wrote: "It's the Jetsons® meet the Flintstones®! The new laparoscopic surgical technique is far removed from surgery as we've known it. Patients are raving about returning to normal, daily activities just three days after their trips to the operating room. Surgeons used to scalpels are getting used to miniature lights, cameras and video monitors. Yet the boldest among them are the steady-handed surgical nurses who have to hold the equipment inside the patient through the tiny incision."

> Robotic arms are replacing those steady-handed nurses these days, but the point of this exercise remains current. Notice the nuances of different types of writing.

Know the Tone of Technical Writing

The tone of the preceding examples is not the tone of a typical technical paper. The tone of this book is conversational, lighter, and more entertaining than the tone of a technical paper. Let's change the tone to give you a good example of *technical* writing.

What is Intensity Modulated Radiation Therapy (IMRT)?

Intensity Modulated Radiation Therapy (IMRT) is an approach to conformal radiation therapy that conforms a high-dose volume to a tumor while restricting dosage to the surrounding structures. In IMRT, the beam intensity is varied across the treatment field. By cross-firing the tumor with multiple beams, the linear accelerator delivers a relatively uniform radiation dose to the tumor, but protects surrounding tissue from high-dose radiation. The certified medical dosimetrist designs computer-based treatment plans; medical physicists perform phantom checks on computer-generated patients to ensure final results. IMRT treatment planning usually requires an inverse process because it is computationally complex.

Time to change the tone again. Did you notice the steady, terse, direct approach in the IMRT example? Did you see a *you* or an *I* in the copy? Do not use *you* or *I* in your technical paper. Write in the active voice, and use the present tense unless describing past events or discoveries. Say, "Doctors at the neonatal intensive care unit are studying the effects of massage therapy on neonates," not, "The effects of massage therapy on neonates are being studied by doctors at the neonatal intensive care unit."

Don't look now, but you've just worked through the worry portion of the writing process. Your treatment plan for blank-white-paper anxiety is going to work.

RESEARCH

Until now, there's been no discussion of outlines. Authors debate the issue, but my opinion is that you cannot expect someone to outline a technical paper before the research has begun. This only adds to the *worry* portion of the equation we've been discussing unless the author is very familiar with his or her topic. The outline for the paper will evolve as your research evolves. As you research, use your mission statement to stay focused on the objective of the paper you are going to write.

Primary Research

Chapter 4 cites primary research conducted by Sandra Gaviola. Primary research is something you have done, not something you have read in another publication. It can include surveys, experiments, or interviews you conduct. What you write will be based upon your own research.

Secondary Research

Secondary research is information that has been written by others. Once upon a time, a discussion about secondary research would have centered on periodicals, newspapers, books, encyclopedias, and video documentaries. Of course, the Internet has dramatically changed the research process. You have instant access to massive amounts of data. There's very little need to pore over musty volumes in the research section of a library. Now, a world of information is just a few keystrokes away. The benefits are obvious; the potential drawbacks, ominous.

Information overload. Reliability. Access. Plagiarism. These and other issues haunt the research process more than ever. Colleges, for example, spend a great deal of time and money working to identify student papers that are nothing more than Internet cut-and-paste assemblies.

PROFESSIONAL GROWTH TIP

Use the Internet to your advantage, to advance the flow of ideas, to innovate, to promote and share the best and brightest ideas for the good of humanity ethically.

Yes, it's a big deal. We have the incredible opportunity to harness the Internet, maximize its benefits, and accomplish great things. Please do so. Take up the challenge. Your wise use of the Internet really can change the world. When you use the Internet to identify secondary research, you are using other people's ideas, inventions, and hard work. Respect their efforts. The process works like this. Read what others have to say, what they have added to the collective wisdom on the subject. Then, when you use their ideas, cite their names (make sure to spell people's names correctly!). Give them credit by paraphrasing their words or using quotation marks when you use their exact words.

Remember when you were asked to write your first few reports in elementary school? Everyone ran to those heavy encyclopedias and copied the information word for word. That's not okay anymore. If you use someone else's words or ideas, you must give her or him credit. If you don't, you are committing plagiarism.

The Internet and Plagiarism

Plagiarism is the act of using someone else's writing, ideas or artwork and claiming them as your own. Plagiarism is illegal and can lead to legal and financial harm to both you and your publisher. Be sure your writing is not identical to the sources you use.

Paraphrasing, the adaptation of another writer's ideas by rewording them creatively, is a method authors use frequently to avoid plagiarism. It is more than just switching words around. When paraphrasing is done well, an idea is changed to convey the special message and meaning you want to convey.

Another method you can use to avoid plagiarism is to document all sources. When quoting other writers or expressing their ideas, be sure to acknowledge the source. A simple footnote represents good scholarship. (*Author's Guide* [Albany, NY: Delmar], p. 31)

The preceding paragraphs explain how to use quotations to attribute ideas to their owners. The material was Delmar's, not mine. When you write, avoid quoting any more than the amount of material that I just quoted.

Penalties for plagiarism are getting tougher as universities and other academic institutions employ sophisticated new software to identify plagiarized or purchased papers. If you plagiarize, you cheat yourself out of an education and an opportunity to learn. Those of us who value the rules and respect the work of others resent it when someone cuts and pastes Internet information to create a paper. Those of us who have spent years of 14- and 16-hour workdays building careers will not tolerate the deliberate theft of our intellectual property.

IMMERSE YOURSELF IN THE TOPIC

Time to assemble your outline. You knew it was coming. Grab your mission statement and research materials.

If you are writing primarily about research that you have conducted, the greatest task will not be to immerse yourself in the topic, but to organize your thoughts about the project. Jump ahead one paragraph to "Writing the Paper in Your Own Words."

If your technical paper is based on secondary research, get into the habit of documenting important ideas or facts on index cards or whatever computer equivalent works for you. Know what you are writing about. Your writing will reflect your confidence.

Writing the Paper in Your Own Words

As you immerse yourself in the topic, think about what you want to communicate and what you would like to know if you were the reader. Here comes that outline. Writing is organized thinking. Avoid overwhelming yourself with information, which can result in rambling, disjointed prose. Can you effectively categorize your information? If you have created index cards or a computer equivalent, use this information to help create your outline.

Jot down five or six key categories. You're on your way to an organized paper. The outline does not have to be a six-page document neatly listing each thought you intend to communicate. The outline functions as a flexible, dynamic tool that works exclusively for you, serving as a roadmap to help you craft the paper. Stay focused on your mission statement and let the outline evolve.

This is an example of a basic outline for a paper on stroke called *Brain Attack Requires Quick Response.*

1. Describe a stroke using a patient's impression of the event.
2. Define stroke in medical terms.
3. Mention limitations of past medical interventions for stroke or brain attack.
4. Discuss new treatment strategies to help stroke patients.
5. Summarize results of new treatment therapies.

Let's take this basic outline to another level. Watch how you can insert thoughts and ideas within the categories, building the blueprint for your paper and organizing your thought process.

1. Describe a stroke using a patient's impression of the event.
   a. Use interview with Mr. Lynch.
   b. Incorporate emergency responder's comments.
   c. "Nothing can describe how terrible it is to wake up and not be able to move."
2. Define stroke in medical terms.
   a. Show magnitude of stroke.
      (1) Stroke is the third leading cause of death in the United States and the leading cause of long-term disability.
      (2) Discuss costs associated with stroke.
   b. There are two kinds of brain attacks.
      (1) Ischemic attacks
      (2) Hemorrhagic attacks
3. Mention limitations of past medical interventions for stroke or brain attack.
   a. Use quote from physician. ("Until recently, medical science hasn't done a good job with regard to brain attacks.")
   b. Outline past practices.
   c. Emphasize slow response time.

4. Discuss new treatment strategies to help stroke patients.
   a. Emphasize new awareness of the need to get help fast.
   b. Use analogy between a brain attack and a heart attack.
   c. Explain tPA.
   d. Highlight information from interview with physician discussing delivery of tPA directly to the brain through intra-arterial catheter.
      (1) Mention physician's credentials; note that he has published more than 70 professional articles.
      (2) Explain the physician's procedure. Use quotes from the interview and from his published papers.
5. Summarize results of new treatment therapies.
   a. Emphasize importance of recognizing symptoms of brain attack.
      (1) List symptoms of brain attack.
   b. Use statistics to show results of new treatment modalities.

Your mission statement and your outline allow you to focus and organize the information uncovered through your research. Notice how the paper is coming together? You've already moved through W, R, and I in the WRITE equation.

THINK, THEN TYPE

With your research, mission statement, and outline as resources, you are ready to write. Find a quiet place, eliminate distractions, relax, and type. Think and type. Get words on paper.

Understand that it can take hours for professional writers to complete one paragraph. Or, it can take minutes. It truly is difficult to predict how much time it will take to put your thoughts on paper. Just write. Don't procrastinate. Don't surf the Internet or start cleaning your desk. Be disciplined. No snack attacks. No fast-food runs. Not for a while, anyway. Devote time to your paper, and you'll be proud of the outcome.

Motivators

Can't get those first few words written? Need a little motivation as you stare at that blank screen or white paper? Kick-starters vary depending on the individual, but here are a few tips that have helped me deliver quality work on schedule.

The biggest motivator is the deadline itself. If the fear of a looming due date isn't enough to get you moving, reconsider your reasons for entering your field.

Another tip is to start in the middle of the paper. No one says that your introductory paragraph has to be written first. It's nice when that happens. I remember a favorite lead of mine: *Five years and three presidencies ago the Equal Rights Amendment was proposed, supposedly dedicated to the proposition that all men and women are created equal.* This take-off on Lincoln's Gettysburg Address set the tone for the article, a high-school editorial. It was a long time ago, but it is memorable because I learned that when the lead comes readily, the entire paper will be easy to write. Typically, however, it is easier to write the body of the article first. You can count on the lead flowing naturally from the content.

Gadgets are sure-fire writers' block-busters. A doctor once told me this, and while the prescription might sound a little too easy, it is inexpensive, quick, and always worth a try. Start writing by hand rather than typing at the computer. Use quirky colored pens, thick markers, even crayons. Or, write on colored paper. Grab a neon yellow sheet and you'll see how fast the ideas start to flow. You'll go back to using the speedy computer once the words start to jump onto the paper faster than your handwriting can keep pace with your ideas.

My favorite weird and wild pens are mini versions of familiar games such as Connect Four® and Operation® . . . which brings me to another helpful hint. Play. Relaxing has great merit. Don't let this be an opportunity to postpone the chore. Don't leave the room and go to the basketball court. Just enter a playful mind-set. Move your mind, lighten up, and you'll dig in and write with renewed vigor.

What inspires you? What gets your thoughts flowing? If standing under the stars or sitting in a dark room or reading inspirational material recharges your batteries, don't delay.

How about listening to yourself talk about the subject of the paper? Turn on a tape recorder. Sometimes the exercise of thinking aloud helps you write. Master this task, and you'll also be ready for computer-aided voice recorders.

Still stuck? Start making a list. This is the technique that I learned when writing advertising headlines. Just fill a paper (or papers!) with ideas. Words. Sentence fragments. You'll hit on a heading that works, then you'll be amazed at how easily the words line up, fall into place, and form coherent thoughts.

Running into the writer's wall can be an opportunity to pause, regroup, and find out what is on the other side of the wall. Is this the end of a page? Look right and left; consider taking a new direction.

You've done your work. You've immersed yourself in the topic. If you are truly lacking the ability to continue writing, you don't have self-confidence. Believing you can do it is as important as doing it.

The Craft of the Draft

Don't worry, just write! That's why we call it a draft. Let these comforting words sink in: avoid pressuring yourself. Technical papers are fact-based. Stick to the facts, be straightforward, and execute your mission statement. You don't have to invent characters, create plots, or rhyme words. You simply have to explain information clearly and concisely.

Get excited about your topic and stay excited. Enthusiasm shows in your prose and helps you achieve your objective of completing a quality paper in a timely manner. Even if you are writing about a new method to cast single-melt titanium into rectangular molds, your objective will be best met if you maintain pep and enthusiasm for the topic.

Drafts? One journalism professor told me that he writes a sentence, works on it until it is perfect, then moves on. Really? That's one bit of wisdom he imparted that I seriously doubt. Do not count on getting it right the first time. Get close. Be realistic. A draft is a first try, a rehearsal.

Here's a quick-read primer on ways to write freshly and communicate well.

- Focus on accuracy.
- Vary sentence and paragraph length. Variety adds interest.
- Less really is best. Trim your prose, then trim again.
- Be direct.
- Avoid jargon. People will not read what they don't understand.
- Limit adjectives and adverbs. Do not over-modify.
- Avoid repeating the same word, especially on the same page. (Three strikes, you're out.)
- Choose active, dynamic verbs.
- Know the rules of grammar before you break the rules of grammar.
- Are you starting every sentence with *the?* Don't.
- Antique words such as *herein* and *wherefore* should rest in peace.
- Do not over-use quotation marks around words to make them seem "special."
- Use a dictionary. Words beginning with *de, non,* and *re* are especially worth looking up.
- It's okay to end a sentence with a preposition.
- Avoid clichés. Find new and better ways to say what you want to say.

EDIT!

Typographical errors (or typos) happen. They should not happen. They are never acceptable, but the best of us still fall victim to a *mispaced leter . . .* or two.

I once wrote a brochure about deploying broadband technology in rural areas of North America. Happily, it was ready for the client in just four days. Because the deadline had been tight, it was a sweet victory to submit the finished manuscript on time and watch it fly through reviews. After it left my hard drive, five people carefully edited the typeset brochure. Before it went to press the artist was asked to prepare 40 copies for a meeting in Canada. No problem. Out the door and over the U.S. boarder they went. Funny thing happened just before the brochures went to press. Someone noticed a bold subhead in the lower left-hand corner that read *Partnershp is key.* Ouch.

Excuses don't cut it. As a student, typos will hurt your grade. As a professional, typos will hurt your credibility.

PROFESSIONAL GROWTH TIP

Edit, edit, edit! Check each paper for readability, grammar, style, and typos, and always have other people edit for you.

So you don't want anyone stepping on your golden words? When you ask someone to edit your writing (and you must), be open to suggestions, changes, or outright criticism.

Sometimes people need to be convinced that they need editorial assistance. I served as senior technical editor on a report that was headed for the U.S. Secretary of Energy. One Ph.D. refused to accept all the edits I had made on the report. The Ph.D. tried to be nice about it; he just didn't tell me that he was not incorporating all the electronic changes I had submitted. I noticed.

The document was in its third draft when we decided to hold a conference call to discuss final changes to the paper. The deadline was two days away. (As it turned out, the Ph.D. drove the document to Washington, D.C., to make the deadline.) During that conference call I went through the document line by line with the Ph.D. and his cohort, explaining my reason for making each change—each comma, each case of nonparallel structure, each dangling participle. I gave him a grammar lesson he probably hasn't forgotten. Sixteen minutes into the conference call the two men interrupted me, saying, "Beth, this is amazing. We really appreciate your time. Now we understand what you were doing and why." Until this moment they had been unwilling to change their golden words. Suddenly, it became clear to them that an editor truly added value to their document, and they became incredibly receptive to my assistance.

Editing is more than searching for typos. Plan to edit the finished product at least five times, and never submit any finished product unless other people have also edited it because fresh eyes will spot items you are apt to miss. (Remember *Partnership?*) As a writer, you begin to see what you expect to see on the paper. You skip a missing word because you anticipate it in the sentence. You lose objectivity as you gain familiarity with the final paper. Ask for editorial help, and instruct your editors to be brutally critical. If they aren't tough, others will be. It's much better for your editors to find problems than for professors, publishers, or clients to discover them.

Steps to Quality Editing

Edit first for readability. Ask yourself if the words make sense. Does the paper communicate well? Are concepts clear? Does the paper accomplish your mission statement? Does your copy make sense when you read it aloud?

When you edit for typos, read backward. No kidding, it works.

When you edit for grammar and style, use a ruler or pen. Move sentence by sentence down each page. Time-consuming? Yes. Worthwhile? Absolutely.

Speaking of time, the best editing tip is to allow yourself a respite between the time you write the paper and the time you undertake the final life-or-death edit. Complete your first five edits, have at least one other person edit the paper, then put the paper aside if there is time. Time spent away from the paper will improve your perspective, allowing you to read with greater clarity.

Use the spell-check feature of your software after each edit. You cannot spell-check often enough. *Warning:* never rely entirely on computerized spell-check (or grammar-check). There are no shortcuts to precise editing.

PROFESSIONAL GROWTH TIP

Egos have a way of getting writers in trouble. Accept editorial help graciously, learn from others, and hone your skill.

Watch for These Common Mistakes

One of the most common mistakes writers make today is trusting computer spell-check and grammar-check features. Don't get me wrong, I think spell-check is the greatest innovation for writers since the printing press. Unfortunately, spell-checkers missed this: *We are on of three international beta sites for the development of next-generation cancer-detection equipment.* Actually, we are *one* of three. See why it takes a person, not a computer, to edit?

Spell-checkers miss words that are spelled *write* but that are inappropriate for the sentence. Here is another: *The hospital will hold its fist health fair today.* First, not *fist*, fits the sentence. However, the spell-checker recognized fist as a properly spelled word.

Repairing Sentences

A 600-page technical document can be easy to edit, and an eight-page manuscript assembled by a techno-wizard who thinks he or she can write can take days to repair. Here are some examples of sentences that needed intensive care.

- Original incorrect sentence: This condition resulted in the chapter on these services to be nonexistent within the original plan.
- Revised sentence: As a result, most plans do not contain chapters on these services.
- Original incorrect sentences: When we begin to recognize industry factors, including market studies indicating that 90 percent of the goods consumer's purchase and the location from which these purchases are made are within ten miles of their residences. It becomes illogical to begin examining more of these "local numbers."
- Revised sentences: Market studies indicate that 90 percent of the goods consumers purchase are made within 10 miles of their residences. Therefore, it is logical to begin examining local statistics.

Say what you mean. For some people, that is difficult. Very often technical documents written by highly educated professionals are difficult to read because of the adroit use of superfluous, extraneous words and the tendency to tack clause upon clause. If a sentence is five or six lines long, ask yourself if you will lose the reader by line four.

PROFESSIONAL GROWTH TIP

Do not muddy your prose. Remember that each sentence should express one thought. No need to cram five ideas into one; use periods as necessary!

Need a grammar guide at your side? You may know a lot about laparoscopic techniques or neurosurgery, but if you can't identify a dangling modifier, if you can't tell *its* from *it's*, if you don't know a thing about commas, your chances of getting your paper published decrease without the help of a good grammar guide or a good technical editor.

I have a few pet peeves. For example, people routinely use *over* when they should use *more than*. No big deal, but cows go *over* the moon. There are not *over* 300 people in the room; there are *more than* 300 people in the room. The *more than* versus *over* issue is moving into extinction. Other, more important rules of grammar are here to stay because they impact the meaning of sentences. Here are the five most common grammar and punctuation mistakes I see among the technical papers that I edit.

1. Periods always go inside quotation marks.
2. Use an apostrophe to show possession (not plurals). For example: *Ninety percent of the goods consumers purchase* is correct because *consumers* is plural. The author of the incorrect sentence used earlier uses *consumer's*, which was wrong because the apostrophe indicates possession.
3. Capitalize only when necessary; do not assign a capital letter just to make a word appear important. Capitalize proper nouns such as April, General Motors, and U.S. Department of Labor. Even if you work at a hospital, do not capitalize the word *hospital* when it stands alone. To do so is to elevate it to the level of a deity. You may capitalize a hospital's name, a proper noun, such as Mercy Hospital.
4. Insert hyphens between two or more words (compound adjectives) that describe the same noun. For example: state-of-the-art technology; grass-root effort; street-level parking.
5. *It's* is a contraction meaning it is. *Its* is the possessive form of it. For example: It's going to rain today. The department is proud of its research.

Proofreader Marks

People who are writing their first technical papers usually get wide-eyed the first time they see the marks that proofreaders make. Chicken scratch? Yes, these slashes, squiggles, and pig-tail delete signs are confusing if you've never seen them before. Look at the Appendix.

You'll have this page dog-eared in no time. It will come in handy when you get papers back from professors or publishers. These proof-reader marks direct you to make specific changes in your copy.

BYLINES AND BLISTERS

Health care advances. Innovative ideas. New technology. The WRITE formula will help you develop technical papers that accurately transmit the results of your research, studies, and hard work. You've earned the blisters for your work; your completed paper will offset some of those long, dedicated hours you spent in the laboratory, library, field, or elsewhere.

Technical work isn't really complete until it has been documented and disseminated. Sharing exciting and worthwhile information through clear, concise writing is satisfying work. It requires time, patience, and diligence, but the personal and professional rewards and the opportunities to extend the body of knowledge about a topic validate the effort. And it feels so good to see your byline.

4

THOSE ROLE MODELS

Sandra Gaviola

WHO ARE THEY ?

BASIC LEADERSHIP QUALITIES
> Personal Traits
> Respect for Others
> Minding Your Manners
> Self-Directed Learning Skills
> Self-Confidence

BELIEVE IN YOURSELF
> Where Do I Begin?
> I Believe in Myself

GENERATING POSITIVE ATTITUDES
> Saying *No* to Negativity
> Being Viewed as a Leader

A SMILE AND A SENSE OF HUMOR

Positive role models have a subtle yet powerful way of moving us. They impress us in ways that are not necessarily easy to distinguish. Just who are these individuals, and what is it that they are doing (or not doing) that we find admirable?

WHO ARE THEY?

In a recent survey (Gaviola, 2002), I asked clinical directors of nursing and other allied health care programs to describe an *ideal* or role-model student. Participants were given a list of 10 forms of positive behavior and then asked to select the ones they regarded as the five most important. Sixty percent of the time, clinical instructors chose peer support as an admirable quality. I was more than pleased to see how this basic act of kindness rated, as I believe we can all use a lesson in offering moral support.

Now we know what those role models are doing, or at least we have distinguished one quality that inspires us: the act of reaching out to others. There are, however, a number of intertwining qualities that contribute to a role-model or leadership personality. Let's begin to unravel the unique qualities that define these subtle, yet powerful individuals.

Former New York City Mayor Rudy Giuliani was recognized for "knowing what to do and say in the unprecedented crisis that struck NYC on Sept. 11." Talk show host Oprah Winfrey was credited with having the ability to "listen and relate," and Secretary of State Colin Powell's "intuitive ability to connect with others" described a man of emotional intelligence (Goleman, 2002, pp. 4–6).

Regardless of the size or nature of your group, someone usually emerges as a positive role model, and is recognized as possessing leadership qualities. Yes, there are "born leaders," but Goleman (2002, pp. 4–6) makes it clear that leadership is learned in life, not in school. He assures us that "if we are weak in leadership skills, we can get better at virtually any point in life with the right effort. But, it takes motivation, a clear idea of what you need to improve and consistent practice."

It is unrealistic to imagine that everyone enrolled in your program will simply rise to the top merely by reading Chapter 4 of this book, although the concept does flatter me. But it *is* possible that you will identify at least one characteristic that you would like to and *believe* that you can develop or enhance.

BASIC LEADERSHIP QUALITIES

Let's look at a list of leadership qualities and remember that your chances of developing them will largely depend on your ability to recognize the need to improve and, of course, a clear idea, motivation, and practice.

• Self-Control
• Ability to Relate Well to Others
• Emotional Intelligence

Personal Traits

Have you ever asked yourself, *Why did I react like that? I lost my temper, I backed down when I had a valid argument, or I felt physically ill because I dwelled on an event that was "over and done with."* These are self-control issues. The ability to control your actions and emotions cannot be under-rated. Self-control is a "set of behaviors which accepts the reality that the only thing in life which you can successfully change and control is yourself" (Messina & Messina, 2003).

Self-Control

Fortunately, there are tools for handling self-control issues. Of course, the list of issues can range from addictions to problems associated with personal relationships. But those are issues that go beyond the scope of our student-related mentoring. The purpose of this section is to help you identify in which areas of your school or work life you need to gain more self-control. Let's begin by looking at a list of behavioral problems that were identified by the participants of the allied health survey (Gaviola, 2002).

• Procrastination
• Lack of confidence
• Avoidance (because of fear of failure)

- Self-esteem
- Dodging responsibility
- Habits (excessive smoking or nail biting)
- Passive personality
- Abrasive personality
- Defensiveness
- Negative attitudes
- The "I" personality (It's not all always about "you")
- Interrupting
- Uncontrolled outbursts

It is time to be insightful. Look at the list and determine the areas in which you believe you are lacking self-control.

Once you've identified the issue(s), then you need to pinpoint which emotions tend to lead you to be more out of control. For instance, if you are an "I" personality or one who interrupts, it is probably the emotion of *excitability* that leads to this form of behavior. At this point, you would have to ask yourself, "Why am I overly excitable?"

If you are defensive, lacking in confidence, afraid of failure, or a passive individual, *fear* may be your emotional weakness. If you are feeling the emotion of *anxiety,* you are more likely to dodge responsibility, become out of control in general (performance anxiety), and experience unnecessary stress from your home or school workload. Finally, *anger* can lead to uncontrolled outbursts or an abrasive personality. Which of these emotions, if any, are causing turbulence in your life?

- Hyperexcitability
- Generalized fear
- Chronic anxiety
- Suppressed rage or anger

Can you see that our uncontrolled behaviors are results of our emotions? Once we've nailed down the emotion that is related to our undesirable behavior, we can ask ourselves these questions:

- How can I contain my excitement?
- Why am I living in fear?
- What causes my generalized anxiety?
- Who or what is making me angry?

Now that we've identified some of the emotions or feelings that lead to out-of-control behavior, it is time for new rational or reality-based and healthy thinking. We need to practice *self-affirmation*.

Self-affirmation is a very simple solution to a very complex set of control issues. Think in these ways:

- I can control myself and my emotions.
- I will take control of my behaviors.
- I am only human and not a perfect being.
- Changing old behaviors takes effort, time, and motivation and I am willing to give of these to gain control of my life.

Finally, decide which self-control issue is your highest priority and then develop a plan and stick with it. Don't become discouraged if you fall into the same old habits. Change takes time. Expect to progress at a slow and steady pace.

If you believe that your needs exceed the simplified explanation offered here, then you are to be congratulated on your insightfulness. Follow through with your instincts. You can start at your facility's counseling office.

Relating Well to Others

Have you heard the expressions "Misery loves company" or "Birds of a feather flock together"? Although the connotation in both is rather negative, the expressions demonstrate the meaning of relating to others. There are far more ways in which individuals can relate on a more positive level. For example, attending the same high school, purchasing the same style of lab coat, driving the same model of automobile, or living in the same dorm are ways in which we can relate to others on an ordinary basis. Politicians work hard at relating to others, especially during the final weeks leading up to the election. Candidates have something for everyone—something that's bound to bring on a smile or a serious wink and a sustained handshake. These political runners appear to relate well to everyone and perhaps that's why we see them as leaders.

In your element (the classroom), role models are equal-opportunity friends and also relate well to just about everyone. According to the clinical instructors surveyed (Gaviola, 2002), leaders in the classroom are usually visible and sociable, and rarely gravitate to a particular clan. They are basically popular and approachable people.

Emotional Intelligence

The term *emotional intelligence* (EI) was first used in 1990 and is sometimes referred to as emotional quotient or emotional literacy. People with emotional intelligence are believed to have well-developed social skills and the ability to relate well to others. They are aware of their feelings as well as the feelings of those around them (Ford-Martin, 2002). Surprisingly, intelligence quotient (IQ) and emotional intelligence are independent. This means that people who are intellectually gifted can be failures as leaders.

PROFESSIONAL GROWTH TIP

Emotional intelligence can be improved with the help of a personal coach/trainer. Material on improving your emotional intelligence is available in major bookstores.

So, you don't have to be extremely intelligent to be a role model or in a leadership position. In fact, being reasonably knowledgeable is simply good enough. The class representative or student of the year is rarely the one with the most impressive grade point average. If representatives are also the head of the class, they were probably elected based on their ability to relate well to others rather than their academic reputation. They usually build good relationships, help resolve conflicts, deal well with change, and set measurable goals. Their competition is personally contained. They offer encouragement and enjoy the accomplishments of others. Now, *that's* an ideal individual.

If you have read this simplified description of EI and believe that it doesn't accurately describe your personality, you're probably short on emotional intelligence. That's okay, you will give those who *are* emotionally intelligent an opportunity to sharpen their skills . . . on you. You will recognize them by the way that they give you your space when you are having a bad day or offer to help when you're locked out of your dorm room.

These individuals are not to be confused with those who create conflict, blame others, gossip, or lack coping skills. This group *needs* a lesson in emotional intelligence. That's fine too. Now, you can hone *your* skills on *them*. *How can I enhance the behavior of others,* you ask? You can start by building good relationships with them.

Respect for Others

There is a simple reason for being good to others: we *should* be. Or we can choose to be good to others for selfish gains, fear of punishment, or not being accepted by classmates or co-workers.

Showing respect for your fellow classmates or co-workers because you feel everyone is simply entitled to it demonstrates a more wholesome, no-strings-attached attitude. Respect means showing regard for the value of someone or something.

We've Come a Long Way

If you are a member of the baby boomer generation, you probably know what I am about to say. If your *parent* is a member of that generation born between the years of 1946 and 1964, ask them to recall landmark discrimination and sexual harassment cases. There is less tolerance today for ethnic, racial, and sexual harassment than there was just 20 years ago. In the twenty-first century, students and workers are protected by federal laws prohibiting acts of disrespect and discrimination. Educational, health care, and corporate institutions can be held accountable for such acts committed by individuals associated with their organization. Claims of sexual harassment or other forms of abuse can be costly to the institution. Your school or employer may have already required you to sign a code of conduct or statement of respect.

Princeton University's *Statement of Respect for Others* underscores the consequences of violating such codes of conduct. Visit http://www.princeton.edu to learn about Princeton University's rights, rules, and responsibilities.

PROFESSIONAL GROWTH TIP

You can show your respect by listening and valuing what others bring into society.

Individuals Matter

He or she has to *earn* my respect. Have you heard anyone say that? *Does* he or does she have to earn respect—or can you be encouraged to value others even when differences in views and backgrounds exist? Individuals, in general, matter and deserve respect. I believe that if you open-mindedly accept the values of others, you will escape the constant internal struggles that are associated with trying to make the whole world obey "your" rules. Remember, not everyone grew up in your household . . . or in your neighborhood, for that matter. We are all different because of our life experiences, and that's that.

Minding Your Manners

This is what respondents to a national survey had to say about America's manners. "You walk around bleating into that cell phone as if you're the only person for blocks. You curse like Madonna on Let-

terman, and your kids think the world is their personal playground."
A full 79 percent surveyed by the research group Public Agenda said
a "lack of respect and courtesy in American society is a serous problem" (Crenson, 2002). People with rude manners and lack of respect
might be the object of entertainment in the cafeteria or break room.
But they may have a bit of a challenge reaching their career goals if
their rough edges are not polished off in time.

Do you remember the student in grade school who was openly
humiliated because of his poor reading skills? At the time it was your
grade school teacher who was responsible for disciplining those who
made fun of your classmate. You are in an adult environment now
and the course curriculum does not allow enough time for a lesson in
manners. Nor should it.

PROFESSIONAL GROWTH TIP

*We'll always be known by the way we treat others. And the way
we treat others will always be a key factor in determining how successful
we become.—Hal Urban (Urban, 2003, p. 67)*

Self-Directed Learning Skills

Role models and leaders might not be at the very top of the academic ladder, but you'll probably find them somewhere on the higher
rungs. Practice self-direction by staying focused on what *you* want to
become. Think on your own, find interesting experiences, and create
your own personal standards rather than following those that are considered to be the norm.

Thinking Outside the Syllabus

As a clinical instructor, I often encouraged my students to randomly
select and read one medical article each night. I assured them that this
would heighten their awareness and enable them to recognize more
terms and concepts as they advanced from the classroom to their clin-

ical rotations. It was exciting to see students enlightening other students with their self-selected reading experiences. I knew the assignment was working when students repeatedly said, *I read that just last night.* In fact, I had a few questions of my own for students who tackled some relatively advanced material.

PROFESSIONAL GROWTH TIP

If you really want to test your limits, spend an evening in the health care library reading and elaborating on an upcoming lesson. Imagine the feelings of surefootedness and satisfaction that you will have knowing, beforehand, where the lesson is going.

PROFESSIONAL GROWTH TIP

If you think that staying ahead is an insurmountable feat, try getting behind.

Eavesdropping in the Hospital?

Of course! Eavesdropping is perfectly acceptable if your purpose in listening is to learn and you do not allow it to distract you from more important matters at hand. Practice taking in all the sounds around you. Listen to the voices of experience. Take mental notes of new terms, debates over patient care, and treatment decisions. We are all on the same team. Our goal is to know as much as possible about the patient and the plan of action.

As the patient describes the events leading up to his or her complete lower extremity paralysis, gingivitis, unaccountable weight loss, or severe shortness of breath, listen, whether interviewing the patient is your assignment or not. This information is just as important to you as it is to the individual who is interviewing the patient. It provides facts and allows you to pass on accurate information to your replacement at the end of the shift. Having to repeat the events that led to hospitalization could cause your patient to feel frustrated and as though caregivers are not working as a team. This is why active listening is in your patient's best interest. And, of course, maintain confidentiality at all times. The consequences of breach of confidentiality can be damaging to you as well as to your patient or client.

The Health Insurance Portability and Accountability Act (HIPAA) is federal legislation that (1) ensures an individual's continuity of coverage (when moving from one health plan to another); (2) increases government authority in many areas of health care fraud; and (3) punishes individuals or organizations that fail to keep patient information confidential (Opus Communications, Inc., 2002).

Learning the nonverbal sounds of your new environment is just as important. Some sounds will be recognized as the "norm" while others will be recognized as triggers for a need to act. Monitors, pneumatic instruments, electronically regulated hospital beds, feeding and intravenous pumps, and radiology equipment are just a few of the "noise makers" you will learn to identify. You will learn which sounds are normal and which sounds require special attention.

Never Missing an Opportunity

Remember that the self-directed learner is always reading, listening to the verbal and nonverbal sounds, and watching. Watching what? Everything!

Don't limit yourself. Look for new learning experiences. Ask for permission to observe special procedures. You will learn which staff members enjoy teaching (this is usually done by active listening). The purpose of your attendance is to *watch*. Save all questions for the most appropriate time, usually at the end of the procedure. Remember that the patient's safety and care come first and that those directly involved should not be distracted during the procedure. Merely observing a new procedure with its specialized instruments, individuals, and techniques is an invaluable opportunity. Think of it in this way: as a new employee, would you rather be the *I'll get it, I know what you need professional* or the *I have no idea what you're talking about* employee?

PROFESSIONAL GROWTH TIP

Knowledge really *is power and so is experience. If you can solve problems or have answers for those who need them* now, *official or not, you are "in charge."*

Employees of health care facilities learn quickly who they can look to for unwavering support. These leaders are generally self-directed learners. They seek knowledge in a number of ways: reading, listening to those with experience, and watching the experts. They are curious about the world around them and it shows. It's hard to miss their sense of self-confidence.

Self-Confidence

Are you aware of your self-worth? Are you self-confident? Having a sense of self-worth is just as necessary to your well-being as it is to your clients' or patients' well-being. Don't hesitate to project a self-confident image. Without a self-confident veneer, your intellect and skills can go unappreciated by those individuals who would be better off realizing them: your patients. Remember, they have a need to feel safe while in your care.

When communicating with your patients, speak with confidence while maintaining eye contact. Accurate or not, one might get the impression that the caregiver who avoids communicating is less prepared or less knowledgeable. It's a bit of a lose-lose situation. The patient does not feel reassured and the caregiver appears incompetent. For this reason, it is important to be assertive, open to communication, and confident in appearance. If you feel that you are lacking in self-confidence, it's not too late to change. Once again, it will take time and lots of practice, but behavioral psychologists remind us that with practice, we are capable of changing our behavior patterns. You can begin by using the following methods.

- Positive Self-Talk
- Positive Visual Imagery

- Self-Direction
- Impressive Nonverbal Behavior

Positive Self-Talk

Most of us face events that challenge our confidence. For example, public speaking, oral exams, and starting an intravenous line for the first time can cause a little anxiety, but don't make every event a crisis by demanding of yourself unreasonably high levels of performance. With meaningful learning and practice you should be able to tackle any assignment or new technical skill with confidence while allowing yourself to say, "I am prepared."

Positive Visual Imagery

Visual imagery is a very powerful tool. I practice this technique often and believe that it is very effective. When you have your first opportunity to speak in front of an audience . . . fast forward. Imagine that your audience was at ease with you because you were relaxed. They listened intently to your every word and felt your enthusiasm. When you misspoke or your props failed, as they sometimes will, you easily recovered with a relaxed smile or a confident laugh. Rehearsing mentally, or using positive visual imagery, should result in a positive finish and an enjoyable experience. (Enjoying the experience is a bonus. Learn more about this in Chapter 5.)

PROFESSIONAL GROWTH TIP

With positive visual imagery, you see a job well done before you've begun.

Self-Direction

Self-confident individuals are *not* full-time followers. They think and act independently and take full responsibility for their actions. They are aware of their surroundings, adapt well to changes, and know where and in what capacity they are needed. They look for opportunities to try new skills, but realize their boundaries as a student or employee.

PROFESSIONAL GROWTH TIP

Think about and then describe the person you want to be and the life and work you want to have in the future. Be specific. Jot down your thoughts on paper and refer to them when you question your career or life goals.

Impressive Nonverbal Behavior

The simplest way to improve your self-confidence is by modifying your nonverbal behavior. It's about your outward appearance. Use erect posture when walking or standing, stand during a confrontation, stand with your toes pointed outward rather than inward, speak at a moderate pace with a strong tone, and smile frequently while maintaining eye contact with those around you.

Quotes
- "Think highly of yourself, for the world takes you at your own estimate."—Author unknown
- "All the extraordinary men I know were extraordinary in their own estimate."—Woodrow Wilson
- "We are valued in this world at the rate we desire to be." —Jean De La Bruyere, seventeenth-century French essayist

---

BELIEVE IN YOURSELF

Do you believe in yourself? Do you have confidence in your abilities? Self-belief is the part of us that is quick to recover in the face of difficulties. People who have self-belief are not easily broken when others say or do hurtful things to them. Their inner confidence sustains them. They move on, not dwelling on or reliving undesirable events. Their self-belief provides strength to move on despite the reality that sometimes unpleasant events have to be faced.

Where Do I Begin?

Others can do things to make us feel good about ourselves. But, ultimately, how we feel about ourselves is directly linked to what we do and what we think. Genuine self-worth is respect that we have to earn from ourselves. So where do you begin? You can start by accepting yourself as a unique individual with unique qualities. Be kind to others, honorable, positive, and productive. Be kind to yourself.

Be good to yourself by doing what you enjoy. Have fun and laugh as often as you can. Be proud of accomplishments, big and small, and don't let them go without self-praise. When your feet touch the floor in the morning, acknowledge your determination and ability to keep going when others might have quit. If you're having an exam or preparing an oral presentation, use positive self-talk. Remember to imagine a job well done before you've begun. Don't be afraid to try new things. In fact, be the first to try! And above all, embrace your uniqueness, no matter what it is. We're all different and that's not going to change any time soon.

I Believe in Myself

"I believe in myself." Can you say those words? When you believe in yourself, you create a self-image that enables you to accomplish your personal goals and allows you to enjoy the journey as you experience one new lesson after another (whether the experiences are good *or* bad). When you accept the highs and lows, you grow to be prepared to take action, whether it is intellectual, social, or physical.

Don't hesitate to try new things. Keep learning. The more you try, the more you'll learn and, as you learn, your confidence to try even greater things will increase.

GENERATING POSITIVE ATTITUDES

Generating positive attitudes doesn't just happen; you have to make it happen. Think about the benefits of becoming enthused. It's a win-win situation. You become more excited about your work and the world around you and your satisfaction at school or in the workplace can positively affect those who attend school or work with you. From where I have stood over the past 15 years, I have seen little tolerance for chronic complainers or people with negative attitudes.

Saying No *to Negativity*

I've worked at a number of hospitals and clinical facilities over the years. My involvement in health care education has allowed me more opportunities to experience interdepartmental dynamics than I might have had otherwise. Anyway, as an outside observer, I can tell you this: most employees gossip about co-workers and complain about management and the working conditions in general. Some gossip is completely validated while some of it is simply a means of venting or perhaps a learned behavior (i.e, everyone does it, therefore it is the thing to do). Is it! I can tell you this: gossip and complaining generate a lot of negative energy and that's not in our best interest. Health care can be sobering and stressful enough on any given day or night. We need the support of our co-workers. We might work side by side as many as 12 to 16 hours. If you're positive and lively, your peers or co-workers will be happy to work with you.

Because we are learning how to become role models, let's ponder that last paragraph. Although gossiping and complaining serve no real purpose and usually cause some interdepartmental conflict, this form of behavior persists. In my traveling experiences, I've also seen individuals who are able to refrain from gossiping and idle complaining and contribute little to pessimistic conversation. When these individuals have something to say, they state it as a matter of fact with no malice intended. When they speak, others listen.

PROFESSIONAL GROWTH TIP

A role model does not gossip or participate in irresponsible or negative antimanagement discussions.

So you see, it's okay to steer clear from gossip sessions and anti-management talk. In this case, silence is often golden. Remember that your comments can be taken out of context or, worse yet, directly out of the break room.

Being Viewed as a Leader

As I pointed out earlier, leadership is not about who's smarter but about qualities we all have or can work on improving. It's about creating that emotional climate in which others feel safe. Hundreds of studies "from religious groups to schools and hospitals have yielded a set of 20 or so abilities that distinguish the best leaders. These abilities shine through in any act of leadership" (Goleman, 2002, pp. 4–6). Assess how the statements below (taken from Goleman's work) pertain to you.

- I know my strengths and weaknesses.
- I deal calmly with stress.
- I deal with changes easily.
- Others say I build and maintain good relationships.
- Others say I helped to develop their abilities.
- Others say I relate well with others.
- Others say I resolve conflicts
- I do not participate in gossip sessions.

Remember Goleman's assurance that good leaders need not be super smart but intelligent enough to understand the issues at hand. He also warned that the "intellectually gifted can be disasters as leaders" (Goleman, 2002, pp. 4–6). Below, is one example in which IQ and leadership abilities are surprisingly independent.

The Biochemist

That's what happened with a brilliant biochemist at a pharmaceutical company who was promoted to head a research team. Some of the habits that had helped him succeed as a biochemist defeated him as a leader. He had held himself to extremely high standards. Now he applied those same unrelenting standards to everyone on his team. Lavish in his criticisms, he never praised people when they did well. Ever impatient, he took over for people at the first sign of a lapse. The result? within months, his team was dispirited, demoralized and failing. (Goleman, 2002, pp. 4–6).

A SMILE AND A SENSE OF HUMOR

Make them laugh. That's what experts on workplace management recommend. Laughter is infectious. We respond more readily to an individual who laughs easily. Maybe we feel assured and safe by their easiness. Your instructor or manager will probably get better performance from you if you feel safe under her or his direction. When you laugh, you are telling people that you are not caught up in anger or feeling anxious but are relaxed and enjoying what you are doing (Johnson, 2003). Do you want to be more creative, focused, and productive? Find something to laugh about.

The results are in. Laughter is essential to your mental health and overall well-being. "The urge to laugh is the lubricant that makes humans higher social beings" (Johnson, 2003, p. 63). If you're funny, get others to laugh. If you're inhibited and seldom find things amusing, get out there and find something funny to laugh about. Go on . . . get going.

Let's take another look at the following leaders: Rudy Giuliani, Oprah Winfrey, and Colin Powell. So what is that subtle yet powerful quality that moves us to place our trust and confidence in their leadership? We really haven't identified a single quality that all role models have and maybe that's the answer: role models are simply unique, confident individuals.

REFERENCES

Crenson, M. (2002, April). Rude awakening; Survey finds manners fleeting in society. *The Associated Press.*

Ford-Martin, P. (2002). Emotional intelligence [electronic version]. Gale Encyclopedia of Psychology.

Gaviola, S. (2002). Allied health survey. Unpublished data.

Goleman, D. (2002, June 16). Could you be a leader? *Parade,* 4–6.

Johnson, S. (2003). Emotion and the brain. *Discover, 24*(4), 62–68.

Messina, J. J., & Messina, C. M. (2003). Tolls for handling control issues: Developing self control. Retrieved March 17, 2003, from http://www.coping.org.

Opus Communications, Inc. (2002). *HIPAA training handbook: An introduction to confidentiality and privacy under HIPAA* [brochure]. Marbelhead, MA.

Urban, H. (2003). *Life's greatest lessons: 20 things that matter* (4th ed.). New York: Simon & Schuster.

Chapter

5

PUBLIC SPEAKING?
NO PROBLEM!

Sandra Gaviola

KNOW YOURSELF

KNOW YOUR AUDIENCE

KNOW YOUR TOPIC—
INSIDE AND OUT

SPEECH PREPARATION
The Introduction
The Body
The Conclusion

PRACTICE MAKES PERFECT

FINE TUNING

IT'S SHOW TIME

SELF-EVALUATION

From the time that we are born we communicate through speech. Understandable or not, we attempt to say something orally. Whether it is ordering a burger in the drive-through or giving a State of the Union address, we communicate often with one another by speaking. *But public speaking? Of course! Why not?*

———

KNOW YOURSELF

One of the first exercises that is taught in theater, the master art of public speaking, is to know yourself and your "Inner I." Like your Inner Child, your Inner I needs understanding and attention. You are all you've got when speaking publicly, and you are the instrument transferring all sounds and messages to your audience. For this reason, it is extremely important that your instrument is polished, taken care of, and respected.

Not everyone is a performer or speaker by trade, some for obvious reasons. However, there is a time in everyone's life when we are stared straight in the face with the reality (as scary as it can be) of speaking in public. So, let's reflect. Assume your favorite relaxed position, or at least a comfortable seat, and take some time to become one with your Inner I. What is your favorite form of communication? Be honest. Is singing, dance, a series of grunts and clicks *your* preferred way to express yourself in public? Whatever your answer is to this question, it will help you to become a better speaker and more in tune with your Inner I.

For example, Julio, a friend of mine, an exceptional painter and puppeteer, had the wonderful idea of incorporating his puppets into his paintings. His idea soon became so popular that every weekend an art opening was offered to him. To kick off each opening, Julio would write, produce, and participate in a puppet show that would introduce the puppets portrayed in his paintings. He would do many of the voices, pulling out all the stops for the show. After the show ended and he came out from behind the curtain, however, he would undergo a dramatic personality transformation. Before his admirers, Julio became nothing short of an awkward rambler.

Standing with his hands in his pockets and his eyes nervously scanning the room, Julio would attempt to make small talk with a fan. So, what's wrong with this master puppeteer? It is simple. His form of communication was not speech. Or was it? He would speak wonderfully and articulately behind the curtain, but standing eye to eye with someone, his demeanor and charm would fade. What did he do about this? He bit the bullet and came out from behind the curtain each night to meet and greet his fans. Soon he had overcome his fear of speaking in public, and now lives happily, mingling and selling more paintings then ever before. Well, maybe not more paintings, but you get the idea.

PROFESSIONAL GROWTH TIP

Any chance that you may have to speak in public, take advantage of the opportunity—even if this opportunity entails making an announcement at a cousin's wedding that a blue '84 Ford has its lights on in the parking lot. These moments are valuable in strengthening your confidence in speaking in public as well as being in front of a group of people.

Along with knowing yourself, it is extremely important to remember to be yourself. If your Inner I can't tell a joke to save your life, resist. Just as it will be obvious that you are fighting your Inner I by telling a joke, it will be just as obvious when you are in touch and confident with your preferred form of communication and, of course, your Inner I. Be yourself.

KNOW YOUR AUDIENCE

Whether it is a room full of executives, a classroom of students, or a waiting room scattered with a handful of concerned family members, each is an audience. In order to better prepare a speech for any audience, it is important to know exactly who your audience is and what they have come to hear. Some questions to ask yourself before preparing a speech:

- Who is the audience?
- What is the audience's age and what kind of message do they best respond to?
- What level of competency does the audience have overall? *Hint:* education level should not be the deciding factor.
- What tone (humorous, straightforward, sarcastic, sympathetic, etc.) is most appropriate for this audience?
- Does the audience *want* to hear my speech, or are they *required* to hear my speech?

Even if you are unsure of exactly who your audience will be, a good rule of thumb is to look at the venue (or location) and the topic of your speech. These clues should give you a fairly good idea of who will be attending your speech.

I recently attended a college graduation. At the ceremony, one of the college's alumni spoke and compared the lifestyles of young adults today to those of the young adults of the Vietnam era. Looking around, the majority of graduates kept a careful eye on their watches while fidgeting in their seats. On the other hand, the parents of the graduates listened attentively to every word.

While this speaker may have been successful and effective for the baby boomers in the audience, he neglected an extremely important audience: the graduates. After four years of lectures, research papers, and pulling all-nighters, the last thing these graduates wanted to hear on their graduation day was some man drone over the unpredictable lifestyles of young adults nowadays.

PROFESSIONAL GROWTH TIP

Each person in your audience is extremely important, and therefore should feel that you are speaking directly to him or her during your speech. If more than one age group is in your audience, take that into consideration and reach a happy medium so all feel welcome.

Here are some suggestions for speaking to a diverse audience:

- Use vocabulary and dialect that everyone can easily understand without the help of a dictionary.
- Speak in relation to today. Not everyone in your audience may be able to relate to 1962, but they can all certainly relate to today.
- Include everyone. If giving a speech on the reasons to buy a specific car, don't give just one example of how the cargo space is good for kids. Include other members of your audience by mentioning how the cargo space is good for such things as groceries, surfboards, and DJ equipment too.

PROFESSIONAL GROWTH TIP

Cogent? *This word means "well-argued" or "convincing."* *But don't use it! Your audience might be baffled or even turned off by your use of "big" words.*

Bring it home. What may help you to personalize your audience is to imagine that you are trying to explain something to your 80-year-old grandmother and your 25-year-old sister at the same time. Of course, this will be difficult, but it is the extreme. If you can successfully explain something to both of them, you can speak to any diverse audience. Keep cultural diversity in mind as well. Members of your audience may not grasp the expressions or clichés that are common to your cultural group.

In case you haven't noticed, knowing your audience is extremely important in deciding how you are going to present your speech. So, who are these people you will be calling your audience? What are they thinking, what do they do for fun, how do they like to receive information? By understanding your audience's psychographics, cultural expressions, and demographics, you are one step closer to reaching your audience effectively on their level.

KNOW YOUR TOPIC—INSIDE AND OUT

Be an expert on your topic. Do enough research that even *you* are convinced that you are an expert on your topic. When researching your topic, make sure to cover all your bases, citing all sources and acknowledging the original speaker or expert. The last thing you need is a plagiarism lawsuit on your hands after delivering a well-received speech. Now I know what you are thinking. *I have two days to become an expert on the early stages of multiple sclerosis? Right, that's going to happen!* But wait, it can. Here's how:

- Set limits on the amount of information that you need to know through your research. Don't waste time on trivial facts such as dates or numbers when writing a speech, unless putting your audience to sleep is your goal.
- Stick to the information that is going to validate your points and make that information fun and exciting for your audience. For example, if you are speaking on the establishment of Wal-Mart, there is no reason to go into detail on the history of retail in America.
- Avoid rambling. Get to the point. Move on. Keep it simple.
- Remember that you can't know everything that there is to know about your topic. Unless you devote your life to one topic, there is no way that you will know everything that there is to know about that topic.
- Simply know enough facts for your audience to gain a solid understanding of your topic.
- Place yourself in the shoes of your audience. Is there anything in the speech that is confusing or doesn't make sense? If you, the speaker, have a question concerning something you say, chances are, so will your audience.
- Don't assume. By now, we all know what assuming does, but we still insist upon doing it. Resist from assuming that people know what a word means or what your topic is all about.

> **PROFESSIONAL GROWTH TIP**
>
> *Be aware of loopholes. If two facts don't add up within your research, double and triple check it.*

So, research, research, research. As tedious as it may seem, it will save you in the end when an audience member has a question or dispute and you are able to support your statement with facts. In the event that you are unable to answer a question, do not lie. Stand on your head, point, and say, *Look, a bird,* or run away screaming before you lie about any facts. You *really* shouldn't do this, but you get the point. Although your audience will understand and respect you even if you are unable to answer a question, it is smart to make every attempt to follow up with an answer.

SPEECH PREPARATION

When preparing a speech, nail down your purpose. If you are unsure of your purpose, it would be in your best interest to find out. That piece of the puzzle will help set the tone for the speech, as well as ensure that the goals and the objectives of the presentation are met. Most speeches fall into at least one of the following categories:

- Informative
- Persuasive
- Descriptive
- Thought-provoking
- Entertaining

The Introduction

Not to scare you, but you have exactly 10 seconds to either wow the audience or leave them in dismay. Therefore, the opening statement of your speech is vital. It should be attention-grabbing, thought-provoking, and, most important, a way to signal the audience to listen up. After all, an expert is speaking. Here are some suggestions for a successful opening:

- Ask a question. Example: How many of you would like to make more money? *Hint:* rhetorical questions work best and discourage that one person in your audience who insists upon screaming an answer out loud.
- Use a quote. Example: Oscar Wilde once said, "Some cause happiness wherever they go; others whenever they go."
- Make a startling statement or fact. Example: Heart disease kills more women per year than all cancers combined. Bet you didn't know that.
- Tell a joke or funny story. But avoid jokes or stories that may be insulting to even one person, or that may be perceived as derogatory. Also, stay clear of hypothetical situations, as they are not as reputable as true stories.

The Body

So you are wrapping up your introduction and you are ready to dive into the meat and potatoes, the nuts and bolts, the brawn and brains behind your speech. Are you ready? Organization is key. The more concise and easy-to-follow the information is, the less likely you will lose even the most clueless of people during your speech. Therefore, a speech plan, or blueprint, is needed to lay the foundation for your speech. Here are some ideas for speech plans suggested by Kathleen German from Miami University and Bruce E. Gronbeck from the University of Iowa in the 14th edition of *Principles of Public Speaking:*

- Chronological patterns. This speech is placed into a time sequence that helps the listener follow along from the beginning to the end of a story. This method works best

with speeches including the history of the evolution of a
product or company or a biography.
- Spatial patterns. Location and direction are used to show
position in this speech. For example, if speaking about
your backpacking trip across the United States you would
start either in the North and end in the South, or vice
versa. This way, the speech is easier to understand and is
more organized.
- Causal patterns. This is a cause-and-effect tactic. This works
best in speeches when you want to give the listener a better
understanding of the relationship between two ideas. For
example, the cause is the decrease of younger population in
Pennsylvania and the effect is less enrollment in schools and
an increased number of retirement centers being built.
- Topical patterns. Breaking a speech on a specific topic into
even more specific sections is an effective way to provide
facts to your audience to digest. Instead of simply rambling
on about yoga, this method allows you to break yoga into
sections such as its history, positions, and alternative
medicine.

Visuals or other forms of media such as Power Point, videos, graphs,
or music may help you to better explain issues within your speech. However, it is extremely important that your visuals do not steal your thun-
der. Your speech should be what your audience remembers. For that
reason, do not rely heavily on your visual aids. Sometimes the worst thing
that might happen, does happen, and your Power Point fails. So be prepared for anything, because anything can and will happen.

PROFESSIONAL GROWTH TIP

*Having prepared a Power Point presentation can be pointless in the event of
a technical catastrophe. Have a backup plan.*

The Conclusion

You want to prepare a solid conclusion. Do not repeat what you have already stated in your speech. Again, the same tactics used in the introduction can be used in the conclusion. However, if you began your speech with a quote, try not to end it with a quote as well. Mix it up a bit.

The relationship that you have established with the audience is winding down and now you need a way to say *good bye,* without having them forget you as soon as you finish your speech. Again, some suggestions from Kathleen German and Bruce E. Gronbeck on effective conclusions are:

- Issue a challenge. Request support or even action from audience by challenging them to take up their civic responsibilities and to make a change.
- Summarize major points. Again, the key word here is *summarize*. Repeating what you said in the speech is redundant and ineffective.
- Use an illustration. Anything from a comic to a photo can be used to illustrate your topic. However, again be sure not to use anything that can be thought of as insulting or derogatory.
- Supply an additional inducement to belief or action. Confused? Let me explain. For example, if you are speaking on cancer, and at the end of the speech you introduce a new, startling fact to the audience, such as you are a cancer survivor, this is an additional inducement to belief or action.
- State a personal intention. By taking this approach, not only are you asking the audience to agree with you and possibly take action, but you are suggesting that you too believe in your message and will take action yourself. This tactic helps gain credibility. Be sincere! If you really have no intentions to help the poor in your community, don't give a personal intention.
- Overall, the conclusion should be presented in the same tone as the rest of the speech.

PRACTICE MAKES PERFECT

Half the work is done, or half of it isn't. Any way you look at it, the speech is written and now needs to be practiced and memorized. Yes, you read that right—*memorized.* While carrying note cards with you during the speech is *not* a faux pas (the wrong thing to do), it is generally best to memorize a speech. Better interaction between you and the audience can take place when the speech is memorized. You will come across as even more of an expert in your topic and a reputable source of information. However, if note cards are needed during your speech, *do not* write the entire speech out; write only the important parts to remember. Sounding as if you are reading your speech is an automatic turnoff. This is your speech, not story time.

Here are some tactics to remember when practicing your speech:

- Memorize your speech. Use whatever method works best for you. Bit by bit or all at once, whatever it takes, memorize your speech.
- Talk out loud to hear yourself speak. It is important to consciously pay attention to the level and tone of your voice. Find a rhythm that flows.
- Record or videotape your speech. Watching yourself on video will allow you to see your flaws before the audience does and gives you time to work on them. Look for things such as playing with your hair, swaying back and forth as you talk, clicking a pen, or anything that might be annoying to the listener.
- Time yourself. Time is of the essence when giving a speech. Most people have only a certain amount of time that they are able to focus. Take that into consideration. Most speeches shouldn't be longer than 15 minutes, unless otherwise stated.
- If possible, practice in a room similar in size to the one where the presentation will be made. The level of intimacy between you and your audience depends on the size of the

room you are speaking in. The size should also be able to tell you roughly how many to expect in your audience.

- Speak slowly. Take your time. You have valuable information to tell. Make sure that you are articulate and that you enunciate your words correctly.

- Take time to breathe. Nervousness and a dry mouth will cause many people to speak faster and swallow words. *Note*: it is acceptable to have water on hand when giving your speech.

- Check the pronunciation of words that you are unsure of. It is better to take two minutes to check the word than risk the embarrassment of mispronunciation.

- Speak slowly in areas that you want the audience to pay the most attention. Have your audience literally on the edge of their seats, anticipating your every word, even if your speech is on the cycle of photosynthesis. By bringing your voice down a level, you will catch a listener off guard while calling attention to the importance of what you are about to say.

- Fluctuate your voice. How many times have you said, *Wow, that monotone speaker was great?* Enough said.

- Do not over-practice. As crazy as this may sound, there may come a time in practicing for your speech where you cross the threshold from being prepared to being obsessed with your speech. Once you are comfortable with your speech, there is no need to practice it as often as you may have had to in the beginning. Twice a day should be adequate. If your speech is over-practiced, it will be apparent to your audience. You want to sound excited, fresh, and nonrobotic when giving a speech, not as if you have memorized it and are just regurgitating the information.

FINE TUNING

The countdown has begun. You are presenting in two hours. All of your work is going to be displayed today. This can either break or make you as the new public speaking idol. No pressure. Just a dry mouth, a throbbing headache, a groggy voice, and wait, what was your first line again? Don't panic. Remember the power of positive imagery?

PROFESSIONAL GROWTH TIP

Before taking your position, visualize a job well done and imagine that your audience was wowed with your presentation.

You have the speech down. Now it's simply time to prepare your voice. Think along the lines of the French language. Whatever is said sounds pleasant. This is what you want to achieve. You want your voice so clear and rhythmic that you could be reciting the alphabet and have people listening to you in amazement.

So, how are you going to achieve this angelic voice? Imagine professional singers or actors and how they prepare their voices before a performance. Likewise, what you have to say is important, and your voice is the only thing that will carry you. Here are some suggestions on preparing your voice, body, and mind before the big speech.

- Wake up at a decent hour. If you are to speak at 9:00 A.M., don't set your alarm for 8:00 A.M. Give yourself enough time for your normal morning routine, and then some. Rushing and being late will not help your cause, or your nerves.
- Do your vowels. Say your vowels, stretching your mouth along with them, *a-e-i-o-u*. This will help in loosening your face, mouth, and voice.
- Sing. Put on your favorite CD and sing along. Take care not to belt the tunes too much; you don't want to strain your voice.
- Move it. You are already singing, you might as well be dancing too. So get up off your feet and dance. This will help increase your heart rate and blood flow to your brain

while decreasing the amount of time you have to think
about your speech. A perfect combination.

- Exercise. If dancing around isn't your thing, try exercising.
  Go for a walk or run or simply head for the gym. Again,
  the goal is increasing your heart rate and blood flow, and
  taking some time away from the speech.

PROFESSIONAL GROWTH TIP

Whether it is a quick jog, a lap around the park, throwing darts, cooking, or whatever else that gets you in touch with yourself—do it. You will feel like a new person, awake, energetic, and ready for your speech.

IT'S SHOW TIME

So you are there. You have made it this far. You have tested your visuals. Power Point is working, the television and VCR are working, and you are ready to go. You are looking out into the crowd. You pay attention to the individuals who will soon be your attentive audience. Don't assume that their level of knowledge is way above yours or that they are perfect in every way. *Nobody's perfect.* Then what are you worried about? Not only do you know what you are talking about, you are an expert on the topic.

Your message will be easier to understand when your nonverbal cues are compatible with your words.

- Avoid holding things in your hands. It is proven by science.
  A speaker with paper, pens, or paper clips in his or her
  hands will play with them and thus will distract and annoy
  the audience. *Note:* if you tend to play with your hair,
  wear it up.
- Avoid using hand gestures. Simply be aware of where your
  hands and arms are at all times. This doesn't mean you

should be motionless like a statue; you may use hand gestures, just not excessively.

- Do not rely on the podium to hold you up—literally. I have seen individuals lean, hug, lay on top, and nothing short of dance with the podium while making a speech. This is extremely distracting and unprofessional.
- Do not pace. It is fine to walk during your speech. *Hint:* be aware of where you are standing when you begin your speech, and stay in that proximity.
- Make eye contact. Nothing is more distracting than a speaker who reads a speech from a sheet of paper. If that's the case, *I can read it myself.*

Remember, all eyes should be on you. Unfortunately, you are competing with cell phones, games, clocks, and what is going on outside of the window. So it is important that you not only be a prepared speaker, but one that can captivate the audience's attention. Your style of dress might be considered here. Below, are some suggestions on how to dress for a speech.

- Avoid plaids, stripes, or harsh prints. I once walked out on a speaker who was wearing a black-and-white striped blouse that was so harsh that it gave me a headache to even look at it.
- Avoid wearing short skirts or other "flattering" outfits. Don't think you can compensate for the lack of content in your speech with your style of dress.
- Avoid shoes that make noise. The last thing that you want is to have your voice competing with your shoes.
- Wear clothes that you are comfortable in. Your clothes should reflect you and who you are. Be comfortable, but maintain professionalism.
- Dress the part. If you are speaking in front of a group of first graders you are obviously going to dress differently than if you are speaking to a group of executives. Consider your

audience and what is appropriate to wear for them. Again, regardless of your audience, maintain professionalism.

• Keep it simple, no matter what the season or occasion. Classic styles and colors, such as navy and white, are always a wise decision when you are unsure of your audience.

SELF-EVALUATION

You have done it! The speech is complete. All of the practicing and preparing has paid off, and now it is time to see how you have scored. Most of the time, the audience will not give you a score sheet in the literal sense, but how you were received and whether or not you will be welcomed back for another speech in the near future should be apparent. Remember that no matter how well you perform, you will win some, and you will lose some too. Don't let this discourage you. Simply know that you have done your best and, like anything else in life, value it as a learning experience and apply what you have learned to the next time you speak in public.

Take notes. What did you notice about your audience? How did they respond to the introduction, your jokes, or you? These are clues that are going to help you to develop a public speaking pattern and rhythm that best suits you and any audience that may come your way.

By evaluating yourself, you will be able to pinpoint your strengths and weaknesses in public speaking, making each time a little less stressful and a little more successful. Here are some questions to ask yourself after the speech. Remember to be honest. But don't dwell on or relive the slip-ups. Acknowledge the areas that need to be fixed and move on.

• If I were to do this speech again, what would I change?
• If I were to do this speech again, what wouldn't I change?
• Did the audience respond well to my stories/jokes/insights?
• What were the audience's facial expressions?

- If I were an audience member, how would I have rated me?

So now you have all the tools to help you prepare for public speaking. Go out and use them. Try them out one at a time. But, learn to use all of them like a master of the craft.

REFERENCE

Gronbeck, B., & German, K. (2000). *Principles of public speaking.* New York: Addison Wesley Longman.

Chapter

6

ENTHUSIASM— SOMETHING HIGHER THAN OURSELVES

Sandra Gaviola

WHAT IS ENTHUSIASM?

THE DEMANDS OF HIGHER EDUCATION

WHY IS MY ENTHUSIASM DWINDLING?
    Pressure
    Overload
    Feeling Alone
    Negative Emotions

WHAT IF I CHOSE THE WRONG PROGRAM?

WHAT TO DO?
    Find Solutions to Problems
       and Take Action
    Set Goals, Then Reexamine
    Learn From the Past
    Take Control of Your Emotions
    Believe in Yourself
    Be Thankful

MAINTAINING THE ENTHUSIASM
    Never Stop Being Active
    Communicate
    Keep Your Eyes on Your Commission
    Keep a Positive Attitude—
       No Matter What
    Surround Yourself With Positive
       People
    Take Time for a Break
    Feel Good About Your Success

MAKING THE TRANSITION
FROM STUDENT TO EMPLOYEE

LACK OF ENTHUSIASM
IN THE WORKPLACE
    Negativity
    Lack of Teamwork
    Poor Management
    Stressed to the Max
    Day In and Day Out
    No Opportunity for Personal Growth
       and Development

GENERATING YOUR OWN
ENTHUSIASM
    Goals
    Active Learning
    Accepting the Challenges
    Communication
    Setting Boundaries
    External Support
    Stress Relief
    Absolutely Positively Positive
    Patience

Enthusiasm is a wonderful thing . . . if and when you have it. Think of the heights you could reach if you had an endless supply of enthusiasm. But what is it and where does it come from?

WHAT IS ENTHUSIASM?

When I think of enthusiasm, I think of energy that comes from within that I need to accomplish my goals. When I am enthused, I feel positively charged and capable of inspiring others to feel the same. If we think about someone full of enthusiasm, or recall the feeling when we ourselves are filled with it, it does almost seem as if we become "possessed" by *something higher than ourselves.* We become intensely focused on what we need to accomplish and set out on a journey with great expectations. We are motivated and in control, feeling as though nothing can sway us from our course.

Barry Farber describes enthusiasm in the article, "In High Spirits," as "the outward manifestation of our inner passion." If enthusiasm is maintained throughout the journey, you may find that the bumps in the road are a little easier to handle and reaching the destination of your goals becomes all the more rewarding (Farber, 2003).

No matter if you're a student, or already working in the health care profession, enthusiasm can be as important as the air we breathe. In each stage of your preparation and working toward your goals positive enthusiasm is healthy and necessary for self-motivation and to drive you forward, advancing toward the goals you have in mind. Likewise, along each stage of your journey, there will be multiple factors that may distract you from your course and diminish your enthusiasm. Let's look at things in perspective, one step at a time.

THE DEMANDS OF HIGHER EDUCATION

The postsecondary or college world is a place completely different from what you ever experienced in high school. Beginning a new course of study can be an exciting experience. All at once you'll be thrown into a mix of new professors, clinical instructors, and students; classes of varying subjects to make you a more well-rounded person; a new environment; opportunities galore for extracurricular activities; and multicultural experiences. You are ready to learn, meet new people, and face the challenges placed in front of you in order to achieve your goals. You are looked upon as an adult, and you feel like an adult. At the start of your new adventure you feel alive with energy, confidence, joy, and excitement. The feelings seem to be coming from within you, almost like an adrenaline rush. This is *enthusiasm*. Unfortunately, your initial enthusiasm doesn't always last until graduation day. Let's look at some factors that can lead to burnout.

WHY IS MY ENTHUSIASM DWINDLING?

The enthusiasm you had initially can suddenly disappear, but it usually diminishes gradually over time due to an accumulation of circumstances. It may occur toward the end of your first year, after your first semester, or even after your first week. Don't worry. The loss of enthusiasm can happen to the best of us at any time or place. The important thing is not to allow this loss to continue to bring you down until you finally spiral into negative feelings, thus affecting your entire game plan you had started off so confidently in to achieve your goals. The key is to catch it early and snap out of it. I'll discuss further how you can do this. Let's first take a look at a few factors that can contribute to student burnout.

- Pressure
- Overload
- Feeling Alone
- Negative Emotions
- Loss of Confidence

Pressure

As a health care student, the amount of pressure placed on you as an individual is unbelievable. You feel pressure from people in every direction all at once. There is pressure to fit in and adapt quickly to a new environment, to make new friends, and—the biggest pressure of all—to get the grades. You may feel the overwhelming stress of having to keep grades high in order to not only keep a scholarship but to stay in your chosen field as well. You may be thinking, *If I fail, I am nothing, I can't work in the profession I want to, or I'll have no future.* That thinking is definitely all wrong. You can take positive action and snap out of it. With all that piled on your shoulders, it isn't hard to see how enthusiasm can dwindle. With numerous pressures mounting, it then becomes easy to slip into overload mode.

Overload

Oh, the feeling of being mentally overloaded! You may feel as though your brain will either explode or have a meltdown if adequate corrective measures are not taken. Who hasn't felt like this at some time in their life? It's as if there's just no more room inside to learn anything else and if you hear another new physics equation or have to figure out one more chemical formula it will be all over. Take a deep breath and look at your workload. You deserve credit for trying to be faithful to numerous responsibilities, taking on a part-time job to help pay for school, and finding time and energy to complete assignments and study for exams. There may be other factors that overload you. Take some time to examine what might be causing you to feel overloaded and ready for burnout. If you're at the edge of burnout or right in the middle of one due to pressures and overload, remember you're not the first and you won't be the last to experience this feeling of doom.

Feeling Alone

There are times when you may feel uncertain and vulnerable. Sometimes not having a much needed shoulder to lean on or a support person who will encourage you and tell you everything's going to be okay can cause your enthusiasm to dwindle. If you allow yourself to get trapped in pressure, overload, and feeling alone, a vicious cycle can develop. More serious negative emotions can arise and accelerate your downward spiral. Find a supportive individual who understands your challenges. This can be another student, or someone who simply wants to see you succeed.

Negative Emotions

If you take no action to help yourself reclaim your mind, negativity can be born and continue to grow. You may become angry at yourself, the world, and life in general. You can become so negative that you lose sight of a positive outcome. Emotions *now* control you. "Research consistently shows that what a person believes translates into behavior" (McDowell, 2002). If you believe the negativity, you become more negative. Can you see how personal negative emotions and negative behaviors can be a huge downfall for you?

PROFESSIONAL GROWTH TIP

Recognize the warning signs of negative emotions and take a break, exchange ideas with your peers, and just have some fun. Return to your work when you're feeling better about yourself.

WHAT IF I CHOSE THE WRONG PROGRAM?

Choosing a program that is not right for you can happen, but it's not the end of the world. I promise. Being in the wrong field can be yet another factor in the loss of enthusiasm. But how do you know if you've made the wrong choice?

Reexamine yourself. Take some time to compare and contrast. Are the factors we discussed (pressure, overload, feeling alone, and negative emotions) at the root of your lost enthusiasm? If you can answer *yes* to this, then you are probably *not* in the wrong field, but just feeling the effects of the factors that cause the lack of enthusiasm. But if these factors or others related to them are not the cause, reexamine further. Does your initial enthusiasm to pursue this major and achieve the goal exist somewhere deep inside of you? Can you recall and still feel that burning desire and passion to learn about the human body and all its functions? Can you still see your "commission" at the end and does it give you feelings of happiness, desire, strength, and focus? Does the thought of becoming a professional in your field still excite you? I hope you can answer *yes* to at least one of those questions. If you did, you are still in the right program.

If you need to investigate even further, conduct more research in your chosen field. Find out more information on future classes and what is expected of you as a student and then out in the workplace upon graduation. Talk to the professionals out in the workplace. Ask them all the questions you have and discuss concerns.

PROFESSIONAL GROWTH TIP

Find out what others went through as a student. Seek advice from diverse people such as professors in your major, the professionals in your chosen career, parents, friends, and fellow students both in and out of the health care discipline.

Volunteer in any spare time at a related clinical site, ask questions, and maybe even get some hands-on experience. Going through these steps and arriving at the conclusion that you did select the right profession is sure to raise your level of enthusiasm.

WHAT TO DO?

Up to this point, we've examined the possible reasons why students lose their initial enthusiasm and ways in which they can find assurance that they've chosen the right program. Now it is time to look at some activities that can get you recharged and on your way.

- Find solutions to problems and take action.
- Set goals, then reexamine.
- Learn from the past.
- Take control of your emotions.
- Believe in yourself.
- Be thankful.

Find Solutions to Problems and Take Action

After you've taken some time to identify problem areas contributing to the loss of enthusiasm, you need to brainstorm a list of possible solutions to those problems. However, it doesn't stop there. The final step is to take action on this solution and carry through to achieve results. Solutions on paper won't fix problems if you don't take any action. Let's look at a few scenarios.

If you're taking too many classes, drop one or two (if this is an option) and remember to plan your workload more carefully for the next semester. Isn't it better to have more time and focus for fewer subjects, to be able to understand what you're learning and get good grades too rather than take as many classes as you can, become extremely exhausted, not understand what you're learning, finish early, but achieve poor grades and have learned very little? You cheat yourself out of a quality education and defeat the purpose of why you are in school.

If certain people are putting added pressure on you, talk to them about it openly. They may not realize they were putting so much pressure on you, and they may have even thought they were only encouraging you. They will usually apologize and try to ease up on the pressure. If you are not specific in how you tell them, how will they know what they are doing to you? If it is your roommate's behavior that is burning you out, again, you *have* to talk to that person about the problem. Together, you can work out solutions to problems or compromise.

PROFESSIONAL GROWTH TIP

Avoiding communication with those who are causing you stress can interfere with your ability to study.

Set Goals, Then Reexamine

Maybe you've started out, thinking you are working toward your goal, graduation, and then a career in health care. While these are main goals to be achieved, there has to be something more along the way. You may never have really taken the time to set smaller, more attainable goals along the way. Now's a great time.

Goals need to be both realistic and attainable. Otherwise, we may never see the fruits of our hard work and be sustained with more enthusiasm to set new, higher goals to achieve. It is initially better to set small, simple goals rather than large ones. Take one day, one exam, one course at a time.

As a student, your ultimate goal is graduation. It may seem far away and unattainable, but it's realistic. The key is to set small goals for yourself along your road to graduation. When you achieve the smaller goals, the joy and inspiration you feel will empower you and give you more motivation and enthusiasm to keep focused on the big "commission"—*graduation*. You then continue to set another goal, then another, until finally you achieve what was once thought unreachable. Remember that your motivational behavior will evolve along the way.

It is also helpful to establish a time frame when setting your goals. If you set a time by which you wish to achieve a goal, it pushes you to work harder and have things organized and finished by a deadline.

If the goal hasn't been achieved by the date you have set, this is the opportunity to reexamine your goals.

Goals are set, but sometimes need to be reexamined after some time to see if we have made progress, still need some time to work on things, or have hit a brick wall and need to try new ideas or take a completely different course of action. Maybe we achieved our goal some time ago and the joy of achievement and the enthusiasm that came with it are starting to fade. It's then time to set a new goal to work toward to reclaim your enthusiasm.

Let's take as an example a patient in the hospital undergoing physical rehabilitation. This patient is required to attain certain goals before he is allowed to go home. After one week, his goals may need reevaluation. Certain possibilities can occur over time: (1) he may have attained his goals and new, higher goals can be set; (2) he has done worse (meaning the goals were either unattainable or he was trying to achieve too much at one time); or (3) he has stayed at the same level, not making any progress toward advancement, but yet not getting any worse in status either. This third possibility may also convey that he just requires some extra time to work at it or may need to find different ways to help him work toward and attain the goals.

Can you see how these principles can also be applied to your life as a student and then after you're out in the workforce?

PROFESSIONAL GROWTH TIP

Take some time to set goals, then question: Are they realistic and attainable? Have you set a realistic time frame? Are you continuing to work on them to the best of your ability actively? And are you working on them in positive ways?

Learn From the Past

No one is perfect, though some may think they are. Everyone makes mistakes and it's okay to do so. It's when we repeat mistakes over and over again that it will become a problem and not allow us to advance. You must take the time to learn from your mistakes and try not to repeat them. For example, you forced yourself to become part of a study group, hoping it would help you understand the material a little better. While this was a great thought and wonderful to try, twice you failed a test miserably. Take a moment to examine what the mistake was and how to rectify the situation. You may learn better independently or with another person (one-on-one), therefore, the study group is not a good idea for you and you should not keep trying to make it work.

Learning not only from mistakes but past positive experiences as well can give you that feeling of enthusiasm because you've learned on your own what works and what doesn't. This aids you in establishing a plan and beginning the hard work toward what you want to accomplish, further advancing you in the direction of your goals.

Take Control of Your Emotions

For many people, this can be the toughest challenge to face and conquer. Emotions affect our minds, which in turn influences both our spirits and physiological changes within our bodies. Some people, known as the "emotionally sensitive," are more strongly affected by emotion than others. Occurrences can make the emotionally sensitive extremely happy or deeply sad. They often take things personally even if someone didn't intend to hurt them. However, you don't have to be emotionally sensitive to have feelings; therefore, certain things may contribute to and play with your emotions, affecting your studies and stifling your enthusiasm.

So often we allow our feelings rather than reason to influence our decisions. While feelings do play a part and are important in certain decisions of life, they shouldn't be the sole judge and jury determining the verdict in your student life.

PROFESSIONAL GROWTH TIP

Remember: you *control your emotions. Don't let them control you.*

Feelings of depression, anxiety, anger, frustration, hate, and fear can consume you completely. These are part of the negative cycle of emotions and will quickly cause burnout. In Cheryl Gilman's book, *Doing Work You Love*, she suggests allowing yourself permission to feel these natural feelings, but giving yourself a time limit—an hour, a day, a weekend, but no more than a week. When your time limit's up, get over it and move on.

"You don't have to make nice or pretend everything's OK or humor others" (Gilman, 2002). But then, stick to your time limit and let it go. If you allow your negative emotions to control you, your path will be rougher, obstacles will be harder to overcome, it will take much longer to reach your destination, or you may not even reach your destination at all.

You are not alone. There is always someone out there ready to help you take back control of your emotions and your life. Talk to counselors, friends, or family members you can confide in. Seek out programs, support groups, or information on campus or in the community. Do research relating to your current situation—knowledge is power.

Believe in Yourself

Again, I emphasize the importance of self-worth. A lot of people may believe in you. While this positive support helps keep up enthusiasm, remember, it won't last long if you don't believe in yourself. If all these people believe in you, and even if it's only one person that believes in you, that's saying something great about who you are. If you feel like there is no one out there who believes in you, I do. You made it this far. You have dreams and want to accomplish things in your life. You would not have made it this far if you didn't have what it takes. Continue to believe in yourself, and the positive characteristics and strengths you possess.

Be Thankful

Sometimes we must learn to be more thankful in life. Many things are unappreciated or taken for granted as we sometimes get caught up in our own stresses and the hustle and bustle of everyday life.

> ## PROFESSIONAL GROWTH TIP
>
> *Thankfulness adds to our positive state of mind, health, and well-being and can open our eyes to what we do possess, what we have accomplished and can achieve, and can give us that renewed enthusiasm to try again.*

My experiences have taught me that it's not only the greater and more obvious things we need to be thankful for, but the little things as well. Take five minutes at the end of every day to jot down what you have to be thankful for in that day. It can be one sentence or several pages. It really opens your eyes and motivates you to keep working toward your goals. There is power in positive thinking.

I've also learned to be thankful for or appreciative of past problems and stresses, because without these, we would not be able to appreciate the good things in life. Even if we don't fully understand them, our past problems and stresses often turn into or are used for good.

MAINTAINING THE ENTHUSIASM

Once you discover the ways in which you can become enthused, you'll want to maintain the feeling, as it will be a great source of energy—energy that not only helps you achieve your goals, but allows you to enjoy life in general.

- Never stop being active.
- Communicate.
- Keep your eyes on your commission.
- Keep a positive attitude—no matter what.
- Surround yourself with positive people.
- Take time for a break.
- Feel good about your success.

Never Stop Being Active

Follow an active learning plan. Continue to take action, working daily toward your goals. Let your enthusiasm give you strength and motivation to do all you can to see results. Activeness can involve research on the Internet or in the library, learning as much as you can about the subject and related areas, formulating solutions to problems and new ideas to try, volunteering time, asking questions, making phone calls, joining clubs related to your interest, studying diligently, and striving to understand the material presented. No matter if it's only five minutes out of your day to read one page relating to your subject, you are actively learning and adding fuel to the fire of enthusiasm.

PROFESSIONAL GROWTH TIP

Your activity, not your passiveness, will keep your enthusiasm burning.

Communicate

Without communication, no one really understands what's going on. Does this sound familiar? There tends to be more assumptions than facts. Emotions can take over and extinguish enthusiasm, as we've already discussed. There needs to be a constant flow of communication between you as student and certain people who are important in the advancement toward your goals, be it professors, parents, supervisors while on clinical placement, roommates, significant others, mental health counselors, or tutors to assist your learning. With the constant occurrence of communication, no one, *especially you*, falls into any negativity traps or vicious cycles. Having open, straightforward communication with others provides understanding.

Keep Your Eyes on Your Commission

Never lose your focus on the end goal. It becomes easy to forget what you were so excited about and are actually working toward as you go through the motions of everyday life and become focused on all the stresses you are trying to take on at once. The factors that dwindle your enthusiasm can quickly accumulate if you let them and you soon forget how initially happy you were. Remind yourself at least once a week what your end prize will be as long as you continue to work hard all the way through the journey. Keep focused on what you must do now in order to advance to the next step forward to the prize. Your enthusiasm will remain strong if you always remember to allow the energy (of your intense focus and happiness of things to come) to remain constant.

PROFESSIONAL GROWTH TIP

Envision how things will be once you have achieved your goal and what a positive difference it will make in your life.

Keep a Positive Attitude—No Matter What

No matter what problems arise, what stresses you encounter, what challenges you face, what sadness you feel, keep a positive attitude within. If you look at the negative things that have occurred as happening for a positive reason, things will be easier to handle and a stronger you will emerge.

No matter what it is weighing heavy upon you, it won't last forever. You have the power, control, and tools necessary to overcome the obstacles. Sometimes it's easier said than done, but it *can* be done. One helpful way to boost a positive attitude is to surround yourself with positive people.

PROFESSIONAL GROWTH TIP

*Human beings can alter their lives by altering their attitudes.—
Norman Vincent Peale (http:www.greatmotivationalquotes.com)*

Surround Yourself With Positive People

You may have heard the saying, *You are the company you keep*. If you constantly hang around with negative people, you will become negative. You will adopt their negative attitudes, behaviors, and energy. Just as positive energy is contagious, so is negative energy. Negative people can drain your energy and enthusiasm for anything and everything. "No matter how strong you are, if you are surrounded by pessimistic people, you will be drawn down their slippery slope. If you can't rid these people from your life, then spend as little time as possible with them and shield yourself from their negative influence" (Farber, 2003, pp. 63–64). Protect yourself—your mind, body, and spirit.

PROFESSIONAL GROWTH TIP

Positive people will continue to motivate you. Their positive energy will keep you positive and full of energy, and allow less time for you to dwell on destructive negative thoughts.

Take Time for a Break

All work and no play can most definitely lead to burnout. Taking study breaks will give your mind a chance to process what you've learned and refresh it for the next session. Make it a point to have some fun on the weekend or whatever night you're free. Have a night without worrying about homework, research papers, difficult subject material, and exams. Set aside relaxation time in the week to ease your mind of stress and rest your body physically. Any amount of time you can give yourself for a break from school and other life stresses will be beneficial. Just remember to do so positively and not go overboard binging on alcohol or participating in other physically or emotionally unhealthy behavior. The purpose is to rest and refresh yourself to keep your enthusiasm burning, not to distract or harm yourself in any way that leads you away from your work and goals.

Feel Good About Your Success

Every time you achieve something good, no matter how small, enjoy it! Smile and give yourself a pat on the back. Remember, it's never too late to start looking back. Even if you purchase supplies for an upcoming project, be proud of your accomplishment. You did something good to advance you farther toward your goal. Barry Farber says that we often get burned out waiting for the "big reward" to drive us farther, but sometimes "the best way to push enthusiasm ahead is to get a series of minor successes going with little activities. Progress alone can generate excitement" (2003). Farber further supports the fact that when one is remaining active, one is compelled to learn and do more as well as work harder.

After maintaining your enthusiasm all the way through college, you've finally made it to the day that seemed an eternity away—graduation day. Enthusiasm is not just something for college students. It is also an essential tool in the real world.

MAKING THE TRANSITION FROM STUDENT TO EMPLOYEE

You did it! You graduated and achieved your goals. You obtained a job in your chosen field and are working daily doing something you love and getting paid for it too. After some time, you may find you've lost the excitement and thrill of going to work and show up only because you have to. Unfortunately, loss of enthusiasm can also happen in the workplace.

LACK OF ENTHUSIASM IN THE WORKPLACE

There are a number of reasons employees lose the passion they once had for the work they do. Here are a few causes:

- Negativity
- Lack of teamwork
- Poor management
- Stressed to the max
- Day in and day out activity
- No opportunity for personal growth and development

Negativity

Negativity always leads to more negativity. As discussed earlier, negative people drain your energy and turn *you* into a negative person. Their negative attitudes and behaviors wear on your spirit. Gossip is included under negativity. We introduced this set of problems in Chapter 4. Some co-workers may feel good about themselves or entertain themselves by slandering others, meddling in private affairs, or learning about and spreading information about others that of course they have no business, right, or just cause to do. Gossip can be immoral and unethical. It is negative and breeds more negativity.

Lack of Teamwork

Unless you are strictly your own boss and working independently from a facility, business, or clinic, teamwork must exist. If you are a health care professional, teamwork is most essential for the quality of care and maximum benefit of the patient/client. In health care the word *team* is multidisciplinary and doesn't just apply to your specialty. In some facilities I have seen and experienced cases where the respiratory therapists work as a team, but consider members of other disciplines as separate entities. Sometimes, the doctors are difficult to reach or don't care to communicate or follow up on their patients receiving therapy. If no one can work together as a team, how is this professional, and how is this of benefit to the patient/client? Moreover, what does this do to you as an individual working in this kind of environment? No good will come from lack of teamwork.

Poor Management

An unfortunate fact is that many managers were never trained to manage others. Many have chosen to take a managerial position because they have seen it as a good way to climb the ladder. If you are not supported, motivated, appreciated, led, or mentored properly by your manager, you and your career will suffer. Even if your department has a great manager, if the top-level management is not doing their job effectively, it will trickle down, affecting your department manager, and in turn, you.

PROFESSIONAL GROWTH TIP

"Your real 'job' is to make your manager successful. Your manager's job is to make you successful too. Without that, neither of you will succeed. Staying in jobs with non-supportive managers can destroy your career" (Gilman, 2002).

Stressed to the Max

Another common enthusiasm killer at work is feeling stressed to the maximum. You may feel your workload is just too heavy, there are never enough hours in the day, you have to bring home work to finish, you're always rushing to meet deadlines and feeling 10 steps behind with every step you take; you're stuck in a rut and your co-workers are unsupportive. By the time you get home you are too exhausted to have a social life or to participate in any physical activity. You're lucky if you can muster the energy to prepare yourself a meal. For this reason, it is wise to learn how to leave your work experiences at work. You deserve your time off away from the workplace. (Your health is discussed in Chapter 9.)

Day In and Day Out

Wake up, go to work, come home, go to bed, and start all over again. Routine. No feeling, no expression, no change. Day after day it's the exact same thing. Nothing excites or motivates you. You go to work because you have to or for the paycheck alone. This is a warning sign of trouble ahead: job dissatisfaction! You've worked too hard to come to this. (Ways to avoid this rut can be found in the section, *Generating Your Own Enthusiasm*.)

No Opportunity for Personal Growth and Development

This is another big cause of job burnout. If you have nothing to work toward, nothing to strive for, no chance to learn new things, develop new skills, or utilize your talents in creative ways and be positively supported for doing so, you will get stuck in a rut and burnout is inevitable. Others in your field will be learning and using great new ideas to better serve clients and become more well-rounded, experienced, and knowledgeable, while you are left behind in the dust, doing the same old thing. When you are encouraged to further your learning and given the opportunity to do so, you are appreciated by your employer, who will acknowledge you as an individual and know that your new growth and knowledge will also benefit the business. When you learn something new that excites you, your enthusiasm for it builds. You continue to feel driven to learn more, use what you have learned, and strive for higher goals.

___

GENERATING YOUR OWN ENTHUSIASM

Enthusiasm-generating factors for students can also apply in the workplace and even to life in general. If you are suffering from job burnout, it's vital to your own health and the future of your career to relight the fire of enthusiasm. Let's discuss some ways to generate your own enthusiasm.

- Goals
- Active Learning

- Accepting the Challenges
- Communication
- Setting Boundaries
- External Support
- Stress Relief
- Absolutely Positively Positive
- Patience

Goals

Begin by setting goals for yourself at work. Remember: *realistic, attainable*, and *within a certain time frame*. Reevaluate goals from time to time and make positive changes as necessary. Always keep your goals in mind and never forget what the prize at the end will be.

Active Learning

Active learning is self-directed learning. Never stop learning. Try to learn something new every day related to and which you can apply in your profession. Be curious. Take continuing education courses, go to the library, visit the Internet, and talk to other professionals in your field. Take advantage of opportunities for personal growth and development offered to you. If your employer doesn't offer you these opportunities, seek out your own. Never stop learning, growing, evolving, exploring, and expanding the possibilities. Learning more and developing an understanding about something you have interest in (on another level) will increase your longing to learn more, utilize the knowledge and skill you gain, and fuel enthusiasm in your career.

Accepting the Challenges

Look upon the huge overwhelming mountain of a challenge as only a small bump along the road to your goal. Formulate a plan, remain positive, and know that you can, one step at a time, one day at a time. Never take on more than you can handle, try your best, and, when you need help, ask for it. The first step is to say *yes* to the challenge. Then, believe in yourself and that you can achieve the goal. Laugh in the face of adversity. Act as if you know the goal will be attained. Out of this accepting and believing, enthusiasm will arise. This in turn will generate more enthusiasm for any future challenges that may arise.

Communication

Without communication, inaccurate assumptions are often made and situations can become worse. How can teamwork exist for the benefit of the client without communication? How will situations change if no one speaks up? In health care, communication between co-workers in your specialty as well as with those involved in achieving the same goals is necessary for quality and continuity of care as well as for a healthy work environment. Remember that communication also involves listening.

PROFESSIONAL GROWTH TIP

Listen, respect, and be open to what others value and have to say as well.

PROFESSIONAL GROWTH TIP

If you have a problem with your manager or a co-worker, ask for a private meeting and discuss specific problems properly. Be prepared to offer possible solutions.

Setting Boundaries

There will be people who come along and feel that you exist only to meet *their* needs and make *them* happy. They will use you, take advantage of you every chance they see, push all your buttons without even trying, and just keep stepping on you. This doesn't have to happen. Establish clear boundaries and maintain them. Allow no one to knock down even one brick of your boundary, otherwise your enthusiasm will be knocked down brick by brick as well. A strong defensive boundary wall from these people and/or their actions will generate and help maintain strong enthusiasm. Gilman (2002) supports the fact of setting boundaries by stating, "Clarify your boundaries. And, no, not everyone will be happy about them. They don't have to be. It's *your* happiness you are working toward. However, if you don't insist on maintaining your boundaries, you will continue to attract people who will overstep them."

External Support

When you're feeling stressed or burned out from work, it's always good to talk about it and not to keep things bottled up inside. You are certain to explode in a negative way later. Find someone you can confide in who is willing to just listen and maybe give advice, but not tell you what to do. Find someone who supports, motivates, and encourages you. You may have one person you turn to for motivation, another who allows you to vent frustrations, and yet another person you feel more comfortable sharing your innermost concerns with. That's fine. Just try to have at least one confidant outside of work; a sister, brother, parent, friend, spiritual director, counselor, cousin, or even grandma. They can give unbiased criticism and advice, and be there sincerely in support and care of *you*.

Stress Relief

It's important to take a break from your work (not during working hours, of course). You must make time for yourself. You need time to refresh and renew body, mind, and spirit. Take moments to enjoy life. Don't let it pass you by. Don't waste your life away for your employer, stressing over matters that are actually trivial in the grand scheme of things. Try your best and do only what you can, but don't take on everything all at once, feel you have to, and then stress over it. Always take time for stress relief, even if you don't feel overwhelmed, because it will generate your enthusiasm and keep you feeling alive, refreshed, and excited, with relaxed confidence. Remember, don't isolate yourself. You are not and should never feel as though you are alone.

Absolutely Positively Positive

An underlying theme throughout this chapter is *Positivity*. Above, within, and underneath all, positivity is the key.

PROFESSIONAL GROWTH TIP

Believe in yourself. Smile, be thankful, avoid negativity, find joy in both little and big things, and allow yourself to have fun.

No matter what, you must remain absolutely positively positive in the face of all adversity and challenges, sadness, and negative people. Practice and train yourself to be able to turn negative situations into positive opportunities, negative thoughts into positive feelings, and negative occurrences into positive learning experiences.

Patience

Patience is a virtue. We often want things to happen immediately, even if we already know it will take time. We want the big "commission" as soon as possible, or problems to be resolved right now. All things of worth take hard work, perseverance, time, and patience, and are worth waiting for. Have patience during your journey to each goal. Have patience with yourself, others, and your environment. Allow things to happen when they happen; it's for a reason. Remaining patient will fuel enthusiasm, eliminating stress, worry, and negativity, thereby allowing you to perform the work at hand with composure and a level approach. The result is quality work and rewarding results.

Enthusiasm is a necessary factor in our motivation to perform well. It helps us to be the best we can be and to work toward goals with confidence and satisfaction. Show your enthusiasm and watch how contagious it can be. Your positive contribution can create an even more positive classroom or workplace environment.

PROFESSIONAL GROWTH TIP

"Fear is living in the past. Worry is living in the future. To be happy, live in the present" (Gilman, 2002).

REFERENCES

Farber, B. (2003, April). In high spirits: How to get yourself and your business fired up from the inside out. *Entrepreneur Magazine*.

Gilman, C. (2002). *Doing work you love: Discovering your purpose and realizing your dreams*. New York: Barnes & Noble Books.

McDowell, J. (2002). *Beyond belief to convictions*. Dallas, TX: Tyndale House Publishers.

Chapter

7

PROFESSIONAL APPEARANCE AND BEHAVIOR

Dianne A. Adams

INVOLVEMENT IN PROFESSIONAL
ORGANIZATIONS

SURVIVAL OF YOUR
PROFESSION: RECRUITING
AND MENTORING

BEHAVING PROFESSIONALLY
WHILE ON PERSONAL TIME

———

First impressions made by the health care professional can be very important. Whether it be during a job interview, patient care, or contact with other health care professionals, your presence will create an opinion of you and your message based on your appearance. How you present yourself to patients and other health care professionals can make a difference in getting cooperation from your patients in regard to their care or in earning respect from your peers and superiors. This includes how well groomed you are as well as your choice of attire. Additionally, when dealing with people who are dependent for their care on someone unfamiliar to them, you should present yourself in a professional manner. Professional appearance must be accompanied by professional behavior. Patient consumers may also judge you by your speech and mannerisms. This chapter discusses the essentials of professional appearance for anyone involved in the delivery of health care.

PROFESSIONAL GROWTH TIP

Evidence exists that health care consumers will judge the quality of medical service they receive based on tangibles such as cleanliness and appearance of employees (Murrow & Murrow, 2002).

PERSONAL HYGIENE

Appearance, whether professional or personal, begins by following the well-known adage that "cleanliness is next to godliness." Through the teachings of the Bible and numerous religious and historical accounts, we have learned the importance of cleanliness and how it affects our daily life. In today's society you are judged by how you appear; hygiene being the foundation for the basis of your appearance. The next step in grooming involves how you modify your appearance in order to keep up with the latest in body fashions.

Many health care employees face the challenge of maintaining a professional appearance without giving up self-expression. Personal hygiene and body makeovers that are conservative and tasteful can transform us into well-groomed professionals. Anything more or less can lead to an unappealing appearance.

The most important things taught to us as children with respect to hygiene is that daily bathing is necessary to remove visible dirt and invisible germs and odors. The same rules still apply: clean skin, hair, and nails are basic to a well-groomed look. The simple practice of cleanliness promotes personal health and minimizes spread of infection. Daily bathing, shampooing, and use of deodorant, although common practice in our society, may not be customary in others. Hospitals and health care facilities usually cover guidelines of personal hygiene with all newly hired employees during orientation sessions so those less accustomed to hygiene practice in our society can be educated and made aware of standard policy.

BODY MAKEOVERS

Remaking of the physical appearance is practiced in just about every society today and has been throughout history. Although makeovers have evolved from using crushed berries and animal fat to paint our faces, today's practice of hair dyes, nail art, skin piercing, tattoos, and cosmetics is not very different from primitive customs of making ourselves more attractive and socially accepted. As a health care professional, you need to base the extent of your body makeovers on providing quality patient care and guaranteeing patient safety.

Hair and Nails

Many organizations define what is acceptable practice for hair and nail fashion. Whether male or female our hair color and style characterize who we are. Hair should be clean and worn so that it does not interfere with our ability to provide patient care. Long hair should be pulled back or kept from falling into your eyes or onto your patients during close patient contact. Today's hair fashion offers a wide variety of colors and cuts. The health care provider should select colors that enhance appearance rather than those that look artificial and extraterrestrial. Males who choose to grow facial hair should keep their mustache and beard neatly trimmed.

Certain areas of the hospital, such as a burn unit or surgical and recovery area, may require that hair coverings be worn. In this case, hair should be completely contained within the cap. Leaving bangs outside the cap or partially covering the head is not acceptable. Nails are expected to be free of dirt and should not be long or sharp enough to tear disposable gloves. Some facilities prohibit health care workers from wearing artificial nails, including tips, wraps, and acrylics.

Health care professionals performing direct patient care must consider the risk involved in the transmission of organisms if gloves cannot provide an adequate barrier due to long, sharp nails. Although it is very common to see health care workers with artificial nails or at the very least nail polish, as a health care professional you should keep in mind what would be considered appropriate for the health care setting.

Body Art and Jewelry

Body art is becoming more accepted in our society today. It has even crossed the gender barrier and is very popular among females as well as males. Tattoos are no longer restricted to male biceps or chests; they are artistically exhibited on female arms, shoulders, ankles, and hands as well as concealed on the hips, derriere, and more intimate locations. Designs have evolved from the wartime heart bearing the word *Mom* or the name of a girlfriend to cultural and even satanic symbols.

In addition to tattoos, body piercing has also crossed the gender gap. It is socially acceptable to see a male wearing an earring today. And, just as tattooing has evolved, so too has body piercing. Today's generation of teens and young adults have adopted the primitive custom of piercing their ear in various locations as well as their tongue, nares, lips, naval, and much more intimate body parts. Again, the health care professional must keep in mind that wearing pierced rings in visible locations on the body must be done in good taste. Also, as with most jewelry worn in the clinical setting, there is the issue of infection control. Jewelry, including piercing rings on any body part, finger and thumb rings, necklaces, or bracelets, may act as a transporter for organisms and therefore promote cross-contamination.

Although little evidence exists about the impact of well-maintained piercings on the management of infection control, most hospitals have a policy that limits the amount of jewelry allowable in the patient care setting to wedding rings, watches, and nondangling earrings. All other jewelry would be considered inappropriate and in violation of hospital policy.

Cosmetics and Fragrances

The application of cosmetics and the use of body fragrance has changed along with style and fashion. Each new generation tends to create their own image through the application of makeup to the eyes, lips, and complexion. Usually, newly created looks are simply an expression of each generation's search for identity and does not cause conflict. Society usually accepts the new look as something that youth will grow out of. However, controversy occurs when these up-to-the-minute images are associated with immoral character.

The patient and the family will get an initial impression of you as a health care professional based on overall appearance within the first seconds after you enter the room. As you move closer to the patient, their focus will move toward your facial appearance. Your eyes, mouth, and expression will send more of a message than the words you speak. Cosmetics, although meant to improve one's appearance and draw attention to unique facial features, can be overdone and actually take away from one's natural beauty. Cosmetics should therefore be applied so they enhance rather than worsen your look. The recently popular *goth* look that many young people wear involves the use of near-black lipsticks, near-white foundation and powder, and heavily darkened eyeliner and mascara. One could compare the look to Dracula's bride. Can you imagine how this would impact patient care? This fashion statement has no place in the health care setting.

PROFESSIONAL GROWTH TIP

Cosmetics, when properly applied, should enhance your natural beauty in an artful way rather than drastically change the appearance of your face.

Perfumes in the health care setting pose a real problem for those patients being treated for breathing disorders or chronic nausea. Many of these patients are sensitive or allergic to or sickened by the fragrance, which further exacerbates their condition. In fact, many hospitals have adopted dress code policies that prohibit all employees who have direct patient contact from using perfumes, colognes, or after-shave lotions. Keep in mind that as a health care professional, you are there to treat and care for patients in need of medical attention; use of cosmetics and fragrances should not interfere with this care or cause further anxiety to your patients.

APPROPRIATE APPAREL

There are several options for selecting appropriate apparel in today's health care settings that are accepted by the health care professional, the hospital, and the patient-consumer alike. These options allow you to exercise some self-expression in what you choose to wear while still maintaining a professional image. As a health care professional, you should keep in mind the importance of patient and public perception when selecting your hospital apparel (Stepanek, 2002). In this section we discuss the appropriateness of the traditional white uniform, hospital scrubs, and lab coats worn over business and casual clothes by health care professionals in a variety of settings.

Hospital Whites

The traditional white uniform worn by nurses and health care providers has been a symbol of professionalism for centuries. The uniform, more than just something to wear to work, commands some authority and respect today. It may even increase patient confidence about the care they receive. Most hospital dress codes today allow the individual to decide if traditional white is for them. Often the choice to wear white is based on the area where you'll be working. In a pediatric unit, young children tend to be more cooperative with health care professionals who do not wear white, while older patients may associate quality health care with the strict, polished appearance of a nurse in a white uniform. There is no doubt that a neatly pressed uniform or lab coat with polished shoes symbolizes cleanliness. What better place to impress with cleanliness and sterility than the health care setting.

Hospital Scrubs

Scrubs are not new to the hospital setting. Surgical scrubs have been part of medicine for decades. Scrubs are the ideal attire because they are made of fabric that withstands repeated washings in hot water and they are designed to be laundered after each wear. Once worn only in surgical suites, scrubs have moved from the operating room to be used throughout the hospital. Although the traditional surgical scrub uniform is still required for the surgical suite or any place where sterility is an issue, the move from sterility to hospital-wide use has led to a change in the design of the scrub uniform itself. Once a solid sanitary color, scrubs are now available in a rainbow of colors and a variety of prints.

Selection should be based upon the area where you primarily work and the type of patients that you care for. In some cases, the department in which you work may require that a specific color be worn. For example, medical laboratory personnel may be required to wear gray scrubs while radiology technicians may be required to wear navy blue ones. This helps identify specific health care departments.

Pediatric caregivers may choose scrub tops in cheerful colors and prints. Cartoon characters and sports patterns are popular with adolescents. Working in an adult long-term care unit is another area where cheerful colors and prints are appropriate. Many adult patients enjoy the variety of dress among their caregivers and they too benefit from a cheery print or a holiday design. Your choice of scrub color and design should not interfere with a professional look.

Scrubs are popular for their ease in laundering and their comfort. This does not mean that they should not be pressed or can be sloppy-looking. In order to maintain a professional image while wearing casual attire such as scrubs be sure to select prints and colors that are not offensive, make sure that your scrub tops are clean and free of wrinkles, and wear shoes that are clean and preferably white. Scrubs allow self-expression and offer comfort but do not forget that this must be paired with professional appearance.

Business and Casual Clothes

Another popular choice for hospital attire is business casual clothing along with a white lab coat. Business casual clothing is a step up from average weekend wear but not as formal as a suit or dress. This type of apparel should still identify you as a professional as long as the clothes are neat and clean and represent a cared-for look. Health care professionals who choose this option may want to wear neatly pressed casual slacks, trousers, or a skirt paired with a neatly pressed blouse or shirt, which gives a somewhat conservative look. Others may choose to pair their slacks or trousers with a cotton polo shirt. The addition of a lab coat will distinguish you as a health care professional. However, do not make the mistake of wearing appropriate business casual clothing and pairing it with a lab coat that is soiled or yellow and wrinkled. Your lab coat should be white, clean, and neatly cared for. Many health care providers, especially home care providers, like this option. Individuals who provide care in the home prefer business casual clothes in this setting because their daily assignment may require them to travel long distances between patients' homes and it may be necessary to go into public restaurants for their meals. Hospital whites and scrubs would be inappropriate in a public eating place. Another concern with business casual wear is infection control. Clothing must be able to withstand washings in water temperatures that will kill bacteria. If you work in an area where soiling with bodily fluids is likely, this may not be the attire of choice.

Lastly, the choice of shoes with this type of attire can vary from clean white sneakers to dress shoes. Make your selection based on comfort first and appropriateness for the hospital setting next. Shoes with high heels or open backs and toes are inappropriate in health care and in many cases against hospital policy. Given the option of wearing business casual will require you to make a distinction between your appearance for the health care environment and your Saturday night style. Bear in mind the importance of your patient's perception. In a study of patients surveyed in California, name badges, white coats, and dress shoes were preferred for male and female doctors (Stepanek, 2002).

PROFESSIONAL GROWTH TIP

A carefully dressed health care professional might convey the image that he or she is meticulous and careful (Stepanek, 2002).

EARNING RESPECT THROUGH PROFESSIONAL BEHAVIOR

There are many rules of behavior that apply to the health care professional while in the workplace. What you may not be aware of are rules of behavior that are often imposed on you during your personal time outside of work. Some of these rules may be formally written in a hospital or departmental policy; others may be unwritten rules that society and the patient-consumer impose upon you. Whether on stage in the workplace or off stage attending to your personal affairs, you are a professional 24–7 (Stepanek, 2002). In this section we address professional behavior within the workplace and why it may influence your personal life.

Professional Behavior in the Workplace

Conduct in your workplace involves more than the technical tasks or skills that you perform and the quality of them. As a professional your professional practice should be at its best. Behaving professionally while delivering service also involves your mannerisms while performing patient-related care, completing patient or departmental record keeping, preparing equipment for patient use, and behavior within the cafeteria, the hospital lobby, elevator, corridors, and even the hospital parking lot. Your conduct includes verbal and nonverbal interaction with patients and family while at the bedside, in conversation with physicians and other medical professionals, or in your relationship with co-workers in your department. How you behave at work is, in part, a result of your personal and professional value systems. Although mentioned as two separate systems, in reality one influences the other. Your conduct in the workplace is a direct reflection of each value system.

Providing Professional Services

Behaving professionally in the health care arena today requires that we see patients as more than those in need of medical care; they are our customers and they expect and deserve quality service. Acknowledging the importance of patients and other clients is a necessary part of health care and your department's role in it. The bottom line is simple: make the customer happy and he or she will utilize your service again. Act as if you own the "business." As a result your "customers" will let others know about the care they received at your facility, thus becoming the best advertising campaign the hospital can buy. Customer satisfaction is necessary to corporate success, and corporate success means job security for you and your profession.

Other attributes that can be added to the list include a courteous demeanor, showing respect for the patient's rights and beliefs, and confidential communication about the patient. It is now a federal law, according to the Health Insurance Portability and Accountability Act (HIPAA) regulations, that patient confidentiality be maintained. Any information shared among health care providers about patient care must be done in a private area where visitors or those not associated with the case can overhear.

PROFESSIONAL GROWTH TIP

Only information relevant to your care of the patient should be discussed.

In many cases, our patients or clients will need and want a health care provider who can show compassion toward them. Compassion can be as easy as listening to a patient's fears or holding her or his hand through a painful or uncomfortable procedure.

A Team of Professionals

Teamwork among health care providers is essential for providing and improving quality care. In Chapter 6 we learned that lack of team approach can break one's spirit. A team of players in any situation, whether it is the Pittsburgh Steelers or the New York Yankees, can expect to win the game only if they work together. Every player knows his role and respects the role of other members. The health care arena is composed of many *players*: dietitians, physical therapists, nurse assistants, medical residents, physicians, medical lab technicians, surgical technologists, and many more. They are all working toward a common goal. That goal, to provide quality service, can be accomplished only if each member of the health care team shows respect for everyone involved in this goal. Too often one member of the team sees her or his role as superior to that of others. Attitudes like this can only cause tension and resentment among the rest of the team and will likely affect the care delivered to the patient.

Keep in mind that you alone do not and could never provide every aspect of care to a patient. It takes a team of professionals to provide nutrition, administer medication, support ventilation, and perform diagnostic testing. I can't imagine any one professional being qualified to provide total care.

> ### PROFESSIONAL GROWTH TIP
>
> *Respect all members of the team and perceive the importance of their roles as equal to your own; it's what being a team player is all about.*

Verbal Expression

Verbal expression refers to more than the words you use; it also refers to how you use them. Appropriate speech involves pronunciation and diction that is learned at infancy and developed throughout adulthood. Your choice of vocabulary is also important. As a health care professional you are used to speaking in technical terms to physicians and co-workers; this is perfectly acceptable and indicates your level of professionalism when speaking to them. But when speaking to patients and their families you must use terms that they can understand. This does not make you less professional; it shows that you have the ability to have your message understood by the receiver. Verbal communication within the health care environment is extremely important for sharing information with physicians, co-workers, and patients. It is so important that hospitals spend a fair amount of time training staff to communicate in a professional manner. Chapter 8 provides guidelines on hospital-based methods of communication.

Telephone etiquette is especially important in any service industry; health care is no exception. Whether conversing over the telephone or face to face, your message will be judged based on its clarity, tone, and choice of words. How you greet the patient-consumer makes a lasting impression about your level of professionalism as well as the quality and level of professionalism of the institution. Your greeting should begin by acknowledging the patient. Say his or her name and then introduce yourself and explain the purpose of your visit. Going one step further, think about how you send your message. Have you spoken in a polite manner or was your message condescending? How you feel about being at the patient's bedside or talking to the family over the telephone is more obvious than you think. You need to do more than simply say the words; you must say them in a way that is courteous and respectful as well as sincere.

Nonverbal Conduct

The unspoken message that you send can sometimes be more powerful than the words you speak. Gestures such as eye contact, facial expression, and posture can send their own message separate from your verbal message. When speaking to your patients or co-workers, make direct eye contact with them. An appropriate facial expression shows you are willing to care for your patient and that you are concerned about her or his health. A smile tells the patient that you mean what you say as you greet him or her. Also be aware of your posture and stance as you enter the room. Do you appear to be in a hurry or anxious about providing care to your patient? The message you send through your gestures and tone of voice should be that you are confident about what you are doing and that you enjoy doing it.

PROFESSIONAL GROWTH TIP

If your verbal and nonverbal messages don't match, the patient is more likely to believe the nonverbal message. Be certain that both messages match when you send them.

PROFESSIONAL BEHAVIOR OUTSIDE THE WORKPLACE

As a professional you will find yourself involved in activities that extend beyond the workplace and after work hours. Often, there is no financial compensation for your time and effort; what drives you is a commitment to your profession. Another part of being a professional is recognizing that professionalism doesn't end when you leave the workplace. This does not mean that you cannot enjoy a personal life; it simply suggests that as a health care professional you are going to be seen as such by the public wherever you are.

INVOLVEMENT IN PROFESSIONAL ORGANIZATIONS

Part of what defines a profession is the establishment of an organization or an association to formulate by-laws, set standards of achievement and conduct, and continuously enlarge its body of knowledge and function. Professional organizations give health care providers of specialty groups the opportunity to discuss current issues, propose solutions, voice concerns about their profession, and explore common interests. These organizations usually sponsor national conferences that offer lectures on the latest developments in the profession. Becoming involved in such an organization can be as easy as obtaining membership or volunteering your services.

Most associations are nationally recognized and many have state chapters that bring the organization directly to you. These organizations rely on the voice of every one of their members to help them define the future of their profession. If becoming a professional is your goal, then membership and participation in your professional association is required.

Most health care providers are first introduced to their professional association while they are students. You may be invited to attend a board meeting or volunteer your services in the state association's activities. At board meetings you can gain a lot of knowledge about the structure of your state chapter: who is the president, who are the other members of the board, what committees are formed, what are the issues at the national, state, and local or district level. You may have to attend several meetings before most of what you hear you really understand, but your time will be well spent if you can take these issues or concerns back to your co-workers and find out how they feel about something that may affect their future.

You can also become involved in the planning of state and local activities for your association. Many state associations form special committees to organize professional conferences that provide educational lectures and activities. This is usually a good place for new members to begin. Together members work to design a conference by seeking speakers on a variety of lecture topics, scheduling breakfasts and luncheons, recruiting vendors, and creatively planning (evening) social activities. Brochures are designed and mailed and conference materials and attendee lists are prepared. Becoming involved in such a task requires commitment and dedication but in the end is very rewarding.

One of the most important functions of a professional organization is keeping the lines of communication open between the national, state, and local levels. Most national organizations provide their members with a monthly journal that brings professional information directly to the individual, such as membership services, feature articles, upcoming conventions, current events, and even classified advertising. Many state organizations also publish a quarterly or biannual newsletter to bring relevant information to the local level. You may choose to volunteer to write an article or become a member of the publications committee to help with editing articles, printing and design, or distribution. Internet communication is now a mainstay for professional organizations. If you enjoy Web site designing or consider your computer skills to be above average, then this type of information sharing may be for you. Volunteer to help keep the site updated or become the Web master and oversee e-mails received or help in establishing a list-serve. Whether it be national journals, state newsletters, or Web sites, your involvement will give your profession another voice.

PROFESSIONAL GROWTH TIP

Becoming involved in your organization's newsletter is just another way to extend your professionalism.

SURVIVAL OF YOUR PROFESSION: RECRUITING AND MENTORING

Today's health care arena has become more competitive than ever (Bunch, 2003). With shortages in nearly every profession, a student considering health care has many options and will most likely opt for the one with the loudest voice. Filling these vacant positions may require your involvement in recruitment of perspective students. Many of you may have gained experience in such activities as students: attending career fairs at high schools, representing your program at college activities, even planning a recruitment event as a senior project.

You may have thought that once you graduated, your involvement in recruitment would end. However, even when filling vacant positions is not crucial, the survival of your profession will still depend on you acting as an advocate for the profession that you have chosen. Keeping a profession alive requires regeneration of personnel, otherwise, as senior professionals retire or others change careers, there will not be anyone to replace them. Regeneration requires that every health care provider be a spokesperson for her or his profession. Recruitment of new members into your profession can be accomplished by volunteering to teach an anatomy class related to your profession at the elementary, middle, or high school level. Become involved in health fairs or offer to speak at community organizations about your profession. Probably the easiest way to recruit is by providing a voice for your profession every single day. Remember, your voice added to the voice of every other member of your profession is what brings new recruits on board and keeps your profession vital.

In addition to recruitment activities that spark a potential student's interest, becoming a mentor to an interested individual can make the difference by introducing a person to a new career to successfully engaging that individual in preparation for the future. Mentoring is probably the most important service you can do for your profession. This requires dedication to the individual and may cost you some time, but it is certainly worth the effort. You can become an unofficial mentor by simply providing any interested individual with the necessary information required to succeed in your field. Or, you may be an official mentor who works closely with an educational program that may refer individuals to you.

PROFESSIONAL GROWTH TIP

When you introduce yourself to a patient or family member be sure to tell them what your profession is.

In either case, mentoring will require you to meet on a regular basis with the individual. You should discuss the profession and educational requirements. Mentoring should also include a period of shadowing, where the individual can observe firsthand what the profession involves by watching you. Your goal should be to keep the student on track and help him or her obtain formal acceptance into an educational program of your profession (Bunch, 2002). The rewards of being a mentor are many, but most important is your example of giving back to your profession.

BEHAVING PROFESSIONALLY WHILE ON PERSONAL TIME

Professional behavior while on personal time does not imply that you are bound to hospital rules and regulations during off-time. What it does refer to is public perception of you outside the health care setting. Those in the general public who are aware of your choice of occupation also view you as such an individual. And although you are entitled to a private lifestyle during your off-time, you must keep in mind the importance of perception by patients and the public (Stepanek, 2002). Off-time includes any time where your actions can be observed and conclusions drawn about you and your profession.

Consider what former patients of yours might think if they observe you engaged in rude or immoral behavior away from your place of employment. They may question your ability and ethics while on the job. In this situation you pose the risk of damaging your professional reputation. Appropriate behavior for any professional should therefore be maintained any time you are in the public eye.

Earning respect through professional appearance can be accomplished by maintaining basic cleanliness and selecting hair and body makeovers that enhance your natural looks. Your selection of jewelry, clothing, and shoes should not prohibit you from self-expression but must not be offensive to those you care for and work with. Making that first impression count requires your attention to hospital policy as well as public perception about your appearance and your behavior. Earning respect through professional behavior requires more than being competent at the skills you were trained to perform. You must incorporate compassion, a courteous demeanor, and respect for your patients while delivering quality care. How you express yourself, through verbal communication and non-verbal behavior such as facial expressions and mannerisms, also impacts the impression you make on your patients and co-workers. Lastly, the most important quality of a true professional is to nurture and guide new members interested in joining her or his profession. Whether on the job or on your own time your appearance and behavior are a reflection of the respect you have for yourself and for your profession.

PROFESSIONAL GROWTH TIP

True professionals will also go the extra mile to promote their occupation at the community level and participate in activities of their professional organization.

REFERENCES

Bunch, D. (2002). It takes a village: Enthusiastic therapists mentor new recruits into the profession. *AARC Times*, 52–56.

Bunch, D. (2003). Investing in respiratory care is everybody's business. *AARC Times*, 26–30.

Murrow, C. A., & Murrow, J. (2002). What makes a good nurse? *Marketing Health Services*, *22*(4), 14–19.

Stepanek, C. (2002). Executive director's column. Making every impression count. *Nebraska Nurse*, *35*(2), 2, 5.

8

INTERVIEWING THE PATIENT

Laura M. Amon

Domestic Violence
Diet, Exercise, and Sleep Patterns
Military History and Travel

SPECIAL CIRCUMSTANCES
The Pediatric Patient
Reporting Suspected Abuse
The Nonverbal Patient/Client
The Verbose Patient/Client
Outside Influences

———

Learning human relations and communication skills is a must when working in a dynamic environment. The hospital and other clinical areas are the "Grand Central Stations" of communication. Getting the message straight the first time is a must, as misinterpretations or failure to gather vital information can result in dangerous outcomes. One area in which information can be exchanged on a very intimate level is a patient interview. This chapter provides general guidelines that will help you conduct an interview in a systematic, intelligent, and open-minded way.

———

GENERAL CONSIDERATIONS

The majority of diagnoses are formulated from the information gathered during a patient interview. Therefore, it is very important to obtain accurate information, but in doing so you must keep in mind the many factors that will affect the accuracy of the information.

In order to get the most accurate information, you will have to conduct each interview in a way that works the best based upon the circumstances. The challenges will be as unique as the individuals themselves. You may feel that at this point in your studies you do not have the skills or clinical knowledge necessary to obtain an accurate history. The key is to listen to your patient. If you ask a patient, *Do you smoke?* and the patient says, *yes,* don't stop there. Ask the patient, *What do you smoke? How much do you smoke? How often? For how many years have you been smoking?* Be sure to follow up any positive answers with more specific questions. A patient usually only tells you what you ask for. Be clear in your questioning. For example, ask the patient, *How much alcohol do you drink a day?*

Talk Is Cheap

There are many advantages to obtaining a patient history. Talk is cheap. Except for the cost of the office visit, it is very affordable to sit down and talk to your patient. Knowing that the majority of diagnoses are made based on the history alone can decrease the number of diagnostic tests that are ordered to arrive at the final diagnosis. Talking with your patient enables you to establish rapport with him or her. You give the impression that you are completely focused on the patient, thus providing healing to the patient. Upon seeing your patients during follow-up visits you are able to determine whether or not they are improving just by sitting down and talking to them. During the history-taking process, you are compiling the "story" of why the patient has come in to seek medical attention. You are receiving a valid report from the patient because it is coming directly from the patient free of outside influences.

PROFESSIONAL GROWTH TIP

Exchanging ideas with your patient enables you to develop rapport. If your patient is comfortable with you, she or he will be more likely to share valuable information during the interviewing process.

Patient Reliability

When planning your interview, keep the issue of unreliability in mind. For example, a patient may be in denial and present with signs that clearly put the patient at risk for a certain disease; an older patient may have a lapse in memory that causes her or him to be unreliable; or an individual who presents with low back pain due to a work-related injury may be malingering to obtain workmen's compensation benefits. With practice, you will be better prepared to question the reliability of each patient. Keep in mind some of the common reasons that patients are unreliable during the interviewing process:

- Denial
- Poor memory
- Desire to maintain workmen's compensation benefits
- Shame (e.g., sexual or drug abuse)
- Lack of interest in personal health
- Fear (i.e., patient may fear consequences if parent or partner learns of patient's health issues)

Avoiding Outside Distractions

Be sure to introduce yourself and free yourself of any distractions. If possible, put your pager on the vibrate mode. When seeing a patient for the first time, the interview should begin in your office with the patient in his or her own clothes. Have the patient put on a gown just prior to the physical examination. Sit down with your patient at eye level or lower to remove the impression of authority. Remove any physical barriers that may be present, such as a privacy curtain.

Your Body Language

The old adage, "actions speak louder than words," is very true when interviewing a patient. Body language can demonstrate if you are open to the patient or if you are too busy and don't have time for the patient. Allow the patient to speak and do not interrupt. It is difficult to instill trust between yourself and the patient in a relatively short period of time; however, paying attention to these details gives the impression that you are solely focused on that patient, which will in turn open up the lines of communication between you and the patient. Open communication will facilitate your obtaining valid information from the patient.

CHIEF COMPLAINT

The chief complaint (CC) is the primary reason the patient is seeking out the practitioner and is documented in the patient's own words. It should always include the duration of the patient's complaint and may begin with an introduction that includes the age, gender, and race of the patient. In order to obtain the chief complaint you should begin with an open-ended question such as, *What brings you in today?* or, *What seems to be the problem?* While patients may bring up more than one complaint, you should help the patient focus on the one problem that is bothering him or her the most.

HISTORY OF PRESENT ILLNESS

The history of present illness (HPI) is a complete description of the patient's chief complaint in chronological order. You need to be thorough with your questions without exhausting the patient. Use terminology that the patient will understand. Listed below are a number of general categories that you need to explore when obtaining the history.

- Characteristic of present complaint
- Location and radiation
- Onset and duration
- Severity
- What seems to relieve the symptoms

PERTINENT STATEMENTS

As you are gathering all of the information keep in mind that if a patient denies having a symptom it is called a *pertinent negative*. If a patient admits to having a symptom it is called a *pertinent positive*. It is just as important to document a pertinent negative as it is to document a pertinent positive. If the patient states that he or she does not consume alcohol, it is charted as "The patient denies alcohol consumption." The term *denies* should not convey a negative connotation. The clinician is merely documenting a patient's response to a specific question.

PROFESSIONAL GROWTH TIP

Typically all pertinent positives are documented at the beginning of the HPI and all pertinent negatives are documented at the end of the HPI.

MEDICATIONS

You may be required to obtain a list of all medications that the patient is currently taking. The list must include prescribed medications, over-the-counter medications, herbs, vitamins, nutritional supplements, and home remedies. For patients on numerous medications it is helpful to request them to bring all of their medications with them to the office visit. Often patients are not exactly sure or even curious as to why they are taking prescribed medication; therefore they may be considered "poor historians." On the other hand, your patient can be an excellent source of information. The amount of information needed at this time of the interview will depend upon the type of services your facility provides. For example, a dentist may be interested in drugs that interfere with clotting while a gynecologist will be focusing on fertility, birth control, or hormone-related medications.

PAST MEDICAL HISTORY

This is the portion of the history where you ask about all of the illnesses the patient has had in the past. It is not advisable to use open-ended questions in this part of the interview. Typically if you ask patients to list the illnesses they have had in the past they will mention only one or two or none at all. It is better to give patients a list of specific illnesses and let them respond to each one. Include hospitalizations (both inpatient and outpatient visits).

FAMILY HISTORY

The family history should include the medical history of first- and second-generation relatives such as the patient's parents and grandparents. If the patient is older, then family history on the patient's children is appropriate. The information you are looking for should include inheritable diseases. Most common would be coronary artery disease, myocardial infarction, sudden cardiac death, diabetes mellitus, and malignancies such as cancer of the lung, breast, prostate, or brain, or lymphoma. Ask the patient the ages of the relatives even if they are deceased. Current age and age of death can provide diagnostic information.

SOCIAL HISTORY

Here you will explore the patient's habits or patterns that can contribute to poor mental or physical health. Below is a list of (socially related) areas of interest.

- Alcohol, Tobacco, and Recreational Drugs
- Gynecological History
- Employment History

- Sexual History
- Domestic Violence
- Diet, Exercise, and Sleep Patterns
- Military History and Travel

Alcohol, Tobacco, and Recreational Drugs

When asking about history of alcohol intake ask the patient if he or she specifically drinks alcohol. Be sure to ask what type of alcohol and how much. Some patients may drink one or two 16-ounce beers per day while another patient may drink a 4-ounce glass of wine on the weekends. If patients state that they rarely drink you should still use a follow-up question to define what they mean by "rarely."

When asking about the use of tobacco be sure to include cigarettes, cigars, pipes, and chewing tobacco. Many patients associate tobacco use only with cigarettes. Ask the patient, *Have you ever smoked cigarettes?* If she or he answers, *yes,* ask how many packs per day and for how many years. This determines a pack-year history. Ask about drug use or misuse in a matter-of-fact manner, regardless of age, race, or gender. No age group, race, or gender is exempt from drug misuse or addiction.

Gynecological History

The gynecological history of female patients is a very important part of the social history. You must document the last menstrual period of any female of childbearing age, especially if you think the patient may need radiological studies. Fetal malformations from radiation are uncommon at standard medical doses of radiation; however, the fetus is most sensitive at eight to 17 weeks of gestation. Nonurgent radiological studies should be avoided during this time. If applicable, the following should be incorporated in this section: all pregnancies, including miscarriages, stillbirths, or living children; date of menarche; menstrual history (i.e., every 28 days with a five- to six-day duration); menopause; hormone replacement therapy; gynecological procedures; date and result of the last pap smear, breast exam, and mammogram.

Employment History

Inquire about and document recent and applicable past employment history. When taking an occupational history you need to ask for a full description of what the job entails, since a job title may not accurately define the patient's day-to-day duties. Ask about the total number of years the patient has worked and if she or he is aware of any risk factors that are/were associated with the work environment.

Sexual History

Begin the sexual history portion of the interview by asking, *Are you sexually active?* If the patient answers, *yes,* then you need to identify behaviors that may put the patient at risk for sexually transmitted diseases, including HIV and unplanned pregnancy, to name a few. Below is a list of follow-up questions that are normally asked by the nurse practitioner, physician's assistant, or medical doctor. *Is/are your partner(s) male or female? How many sexual partners have you had? Are you married? Do you use protection?* It is also important to ask the patient if he or she is in a monogamous relationship. Patients will have different definitions of monogamy. The true definition of monogamy is "the marriage of mating system in which each partner has but one mate" (Stedmen, 2001). Many patients define monogamy as being with one sexual partner at a time as opposed to being with only one sexual partner in a lifetime.

PROFESSIONAL GROWTH TIP

When obtaining the sexual history do not assume that the age of the patient relates to the patient's sexual activity. Older individuals as well as preadolescents engage in sexual activity.

Domestic Violence

In February 2002, a Primary Care study in the *British Medical Journal* stated that screening for domestic violence identifies a history of domestic violence in more than 40 percent of women seen in general practice with a particularly high risk for pregnant women (Richardson et al., 2002). Many victims will not freely give you information about the abuse so you need to ask direct questions in a nonaccusatory manner. Since domestic violence is common, specific questions should be asked about it routinely. For example: At any time, has your partner (male or female) hit, kicked, or otherwise hurt or frightened you? Encourage the patient to talk about the situation. Frequently the perpetrator is with the victim so if anyone has accompanied the patient, that person should be asked to leave.

Diet, Exercise, and Sleep Patterns

A patient's diet, exercise habits, and sleep patterns will indicate whether or not the patient is aware of her or his health. Patients who eat healthful foods tend to lead healthier lives in general and practice better hygiene. On the contrary, patients who consume a diet high in fat and sugar are more prone to weight gain and elevated cholesterol levels and are at an increased risk of developing life-threatening diseases such as diabetes, heart disease, and stroke. Poor dietary habits often correlate with a sedentary lifestyle. Lack of exercise can lead to heart disease, poor circulation, osteoporosis, weight gain, high cholesterol, and depression.

PROFESSIONAL GROWTH TIP

Encouraging your patients to incorporate exercise into their daily routine can help them enjoy an extended and improved quality of life.

The majority of adults require about eight hours of sleep per night in order to feel rested and fully alert the next day. Patients who have trouble falling asleep may be experiencing symptoms of anxiety while patients who wake up early in the morning (3:00 or 4:00 A.M.) may be experiencing symptoms of depression or menopause. Inquiring about diet, exercise, sleep patterns, or even hobbies with your patients will provide you with insight into their activities of daily living and help you discover the type of patient you are tending to.

Military History and Travel

Asking a patient about recent travel including any recent military work is important in identifying patient exposure to less common diseases that you might not think about. Patients who travel to emerging nations may be exposed to malaria, yellow fever, dengue fever, or other diseases.

SPECIAL CIRCUMSTANCES

Special circumstances can be more of the rule than the exception. Special circumstances range from the uncooperative pediatric patient to the controlling partner. You will have to be an astute observer and learn to handle each circumstance appropriately.

- The Pediatric Patient
- Reporting Suspected Abuse
- The Nonverbal Patient/Client
- The Verbose Patient
- Outside Influences

The Pediatric Patient

Communicating with pediatric patients requires a different approach. Depending on the patient's age you may be communicating primarily with the parent than with the infant/toddler/child patient. Maternal and paternal history is just as important as the pediatric patient's history; therefore, it is necessary to interview the parents or informed guardians of a pediatric patient.

PROFESSIONAL GROWTH TIP

When obtaining information about an infant or small child, it is best to keep the child in the parent's or guardian's lap.

There is no need to initially place the infant/small child on the examining table until it is absolutely necessary. You will obtain more information if the child is kept quiet in the parent's or guardian's lap or playing with some toys. You will also be able to observe the interaction between the adult and child and actually see some of the physical and emotional developmental milestones the patient has achieved.

It is very important to determine the immunizations that the pediatric patient has received. Immunizations are an essential part of well-child care. Always ask if the patient had any reactions to prior immunizations before administering any further ones. Inquire about common childhood illnesses such as chicken pox, measles, mumps, rubella, frequent sore throats, or frequent ear infections. In older children it is important to ask about school performance and extracurricular activities. The family dynamics (nuclear versus blended) as well as the child's emotional experiences at school should be documented and examined further if necessary.

PROFESSIONAL GROWTH TIP

Include in your pediatric interview the following questions: Do you live with both of your parents? Do both parents work outside the home? Do you have any siblings?

Reporting Suspected Abuse

Reporting child abuse when you suspect it and did not witness the actual abuse is a daunting task for all health care practitioners. A journal article from the *American Family Physician* in January 2002 states that "all 50 states have passed some form of legislation mandating that professionals who come into contact with children report any suspected abuse" (Gandle, 2002). Some states go further and state that "any person" who suspects child abuse should report it. It is imperative that you know your state requirements. The Child Abuse Prevention and Treatment Act has required all states to "enact legislation providing that reporters of suspected abuse are exempt from prosecution" (Gandle, 2002). This is to protect you from criminal and/or civil liability in the case that you have reported the suspected abuse in "good faith" regardless of the outcome.

The Nonverbal Patient/Client

At times you may be required to give a treatment or perform a test on a patient who is unable to speak to you. In those cases you can ascertain information from the medical chart, hospital staff, or family members. Before providing any treatment be sure to confirm the patient's identity by checking the hospital identification bracelet.

The Verbose Patient/Client

You may encounter a patient who is talking too much, making it difficult to obtain a history in a timely, organized fashion. It can be very difficult to tell patients that they are talking too much or even to ask them to use brief responses. You may want to multitask. For example, you may want to set up an instrument tray or gather equipment while maintaining frequent eye contact with the patient.

Outside Influences

Outside influences may affect your ability to obtain an accurate and valid report from the patient. You may be interviewing a female patient who brings along her boyfriend who is answering all of the questions for the patient. You may ask the boyfriend to refrain from answering the questions directed at the patient or even ask him to leave the room. This situation is also common with parents and adolescents. An adolescent patient may not be as honest in answering the questions when a parent is in the room. You may want to consider making it a policy to initially interview each of your patients alone and then invite any accompanying family member or friends into the room with the patient's permission at the end of the visit.

PROFESSIONAL GROWTH TIP

If outside influence occurs in your office, establish a policy that each patient is interviewed alone. This will prevent individuals from feeling as though they are being singled out.

For a student, the art of interviewing a patient can be overwhelming. You may feel uneasy with the fact that you are "prying" into a patient's private matters and revealing information about someone with whom you do not have a relationship. Because you are a student you are keenly aware of this. You should proceed cautiously with your patients, treat them with the utmost respect, and never forget these feelings as you become more experienced.

REFERENCES

Gandle, E. L. (2002). It sounds like child abuse—but is it? *American Family Physician, 65*(2). Retrieved January from http://www.mdconsult.com.

Richardson, J., et al. (2002). Primary care study. *British Medical Journal, 324*–374.

Stedmen's Medical Dictionary (27th ed.). (2001). New York: Lippincott Williams & Wilkins.

Chapter

9

WHAT ABOUT
MY HEALTH?

Sandra Gaviola

THE MIND AND BODY
RELATIONSHIP
    Harmful Effects of Naturally
        Occurring Chemicals
    Bringing on the Effects of
        Your Feel-Good Chemicals
    The Choice Is Mine!

PHYSICAL ACTIVITIES THAT CREATE
A HEALTHY MIND AND BODY
    Walking
    Running
    Strength Training
    Stretching

EMOTIONAL HABITS THAT CREATE
A HEALTHY MIND AND BODY
    Learn to Relax by Meditating
    Build Friendships
    Do Things That Healthy Individuals Do
    Don't Dwell
    Set Yourself Up for Success
    Laugh a Lot!

AVOIDING YOUR OWN
HEALTH CRISIS
Shift Work
Food Binging
Alcohol Abuse
Cigarette Smoking
Prescription Drug Misuse
Ecstasy, Heroin, and Speed

———

You must be a caring person. You are pursuing a career that is based on helping others improve or maintain their health. The health care profession can challenge your resilience, so you must promise to pay special attention to your personal needs in the years ahead. Using some very simple, timesaving, and inexpensive ways to attain optimal emotional and physical health will create a more energetic and confident you. Let's look at some ways in which you can begin right now, even with a busy school or work schedule.

I think that my 70-year-old father believes he is still in his 40s. He thinks and acts like a younger man. His posture is relaxed. He is energetic, positive, and still has a great sense of humor. He genuinely enjoys laughter. I believe his body responds to his mind . . . *or* . . . does his mind respond to his body? Is his life on a continually even keel? Not at all. Does he handle adversities and other sources of stress in positive ways? Absolutely. He stays physically active, doing the things that he enjoys. For him, exercise is not hard work at all. He finds pleasure in walking a few blocks to chat with friends or shovel snow from their walkways. He eats what is good for him, reads to relax, has a regular sleep pattern, and begins every morning with a moment of meditation.

I know you are a very busy student or a new graduate with personal responsibilities beyond those of a 70-year-old retired man. But my father didn't begin a new routine the year he retired from his full-time job. My father practiced the same healthy habits 40 years ago. This *is* the time for you to learn how to be good to your mind and body. You will be rewarded almost instantly with a sense of overall well-being. You will also learn that living well has never been so easy!

THE MIND AND BODY RELATIONSHIP

When I think of my father and others like him, It's difficult to imagine a healthy mind without a healthy body and vice versa. It's as if the mind and body are intimately related. And they are.

Dr. David Spiegel, director of Stanford's Psychosocial Treatment Laboratory, cites a study of patients with psoriasis in which half practiced meditation and the other half didn't; the first group healed faster. Other studies show that "patients who are part of a rich social network have lower levels of disease-causing hormones than loners, that people who pray regularly tend to live longer and that breast-cancer patients who have an optimistic attitude or an ability to express anger about their disease tend to live somewhat longer than those who don't" (Lemonic, 2003, p. 69). These studies suggest that our behavior and attitudes can directly impact our physical well-being.

Your body is virtually one big "package" of chemicals. You may already know that. What you may not know is that you are capable of *minimizing* the disease-causing chemicals from flooding throughout your body as well as *enhancing* the surge of "feel-good" chemicals. We will elaborate on some of these naturally occurring hormones and neurotransmitters (chemical substances that carry information along a nerve pathway) in this chapter.

There is probably no better time than right now for you to learn about these hormones and neurotransmitters and how their levels can be either disease-causing or mood-enhancing.

Harmful Effects of Naturally Occurring Chemicals

You are probably familiar with the "fight or flight" response. This effect is explained by a sudden release of chemicals into the bloodstream when an individual is in immediate danger. These chemicals create changes in the body that prepare you for immediate mental and physical lifesaving action. If the fight or flight response is short-lived (i.e., an unexpected knock at the door or a 15-minute public speaking assignment), the chemicals released can be beneficial. This is considered *acute stress.* Under long-term or *chronic stress* (i.e., facing continual deadlines, trading sleep for schoolwork, or coping with a turbulent relationship), the same chemicals can cause a number of life-threatening diseases.

For the purpose of disease prevention, let's concentrate on the effects of *sustained* levels of stress-related elements in the circulation. Stress begins in the brain. When you encounter a threatening event, structures within the brain detect trouble ahead and direct glands to release chemicals and nerve impulses to various organs of the body to prepare for fight or flight. This sequence of events can be a lifesaving physiological response. On the other hand, a sustained response (associated with chronic stress) can be life-threatening. Notice the harmful effects of these "lifesaving" substances.

- Adrenaline (epinephrine)
- Cortisol
- Glucocorticoids
- Noradrenaline (norepinephrine)

Adrenaline: Released by the adrenal glands, adrenaline makes your heart pump faster and your lungs exchange gases more efficiently to supply the body with oxygen. Adrenaline also raises the level of insulin, increasing your appetite.
Harmful effects: High blood pressure, cardiac irritability, and obesity (linked to diabetes, heart disease, and several types of cancers). Long-term exposure can cause damage to your arteries.

Cortisol: A steroid hormone that occurs naturally in the body, cortisol increases your appetite for huge quantities of sweets and carbohydrates that provide you with energy.

Harmful effects: Obesity (linked to diabetes, heart disease, and several types of cancers). Long-term exposure can weaken your immune system.

Glucocorticoids: Also released by the adrenal glands, glucocorticoids help your body convert sugar into energy.
Harmful effects: Under chronic stress, low levels of glucocorticoids remain in circulation, leading to a weakened immune system, osteoporosis, and even memory problems.

Noradrenaline: Released by nerve cells, this chemical excites the heart muscle, tenses other muscles, and improves alertness and wakefulness.
Harmful effects: High blood pressure, cardiac irritability, and emotional agitation.

Not *all* environmentally or psychologically related chemical release is harmful. In fact, positive physical activity as well as the process of thinking happy thoughts can create a surge of mood-enhancing and stress-reducing chemicals. Throughout this chapter you will learn how to prevent stress-related diseases by becoming more mindful and improving your emotional and physical habits.

Bringing on the Effects of Your Feel-Good Chemicals

The best things in life truly are free! Mood-enhancing chemicals are produced by the body and there are ways you can prompt their release into your bloodstream. Have you ever heard of "runner's high"? Some antidepressant drugs work by keeping naturally occurring chemicals present in the brain for a prolonged period of time. Do you recognize any of these naturally occurring mood-enhancing chemicals?

- Endorphins
- Dopamine
- Serotonin
- Oxytocin

There's strong evidence that moderate exercise—a brisk walk or a weight training session—triggers the release of "pleasure chemicals" known as endorphins. And the "feel-good" chemicals, dopamine and serotonin (found in the brain), can reduce depression when activated by working up a good sweat.

Endorphins: Endorphins are naturally occurring opiates that increase pleasure and reduce pain. A long-distance runner, a woman giving birth, and a person in shock after a car wreck all have elevated levels of endorphins.
Benefits: Increases your pleasure and decreases your perception of pain.

Dopamine: Dopamine helps control voluntary movement and causes cerebral arteries to dilate, increasing blood flow to the brain. The presence of this chemical helps you to react and think quickly.
Benefits: Relieves symptoms of depression.

Serotonin: Serotonin is involved in the regulation of sleep and linked to mood.
Benefits: Makes you sleepy and reduces the need for you to be in control.

Oxytocin: In humans, oxytocin is released in response to intense emotional states. It is released during sexual orgasm in both men and women.
Benefits: Counteracts stress and produces a calming effect. Influences our ability to bond well with others.

The Choice Is Mine!

Knowing the health *risks* associated with long-term stress and the *benefits* of moderate exercise, do you feel capable of making some lifestyle changes? Together, an exercise plan, stress management, weight control, and a healthy lifestyle can help you feel more confident and energetic, and allow you to enjoy the benefits of a healthy body. The choice is yours!

PHYSICAL ACTIVITIES THAT CREATE A HEALTHY MIND AND BODY

In addition to numerous remedies for stress and the blues, "exercise has become an appealing new alternative to alter one's mood" (Husseini, 2003). Remember, my father didn't think twice before taking a brisk walk down the city sidewalks where he found a number of pleasurable activities along the way. He only walked to get there. His ultimate satisfaction was in connecting with friends, being outside, and helping others. I don't think that my father was aware of the physiological benefits of walking, building strong friendships, or being in the sun's light. But the benefits showed. He was and still is an emotionally and physically fit man.

The best activities are the ones that you enjoy. If you feel inconvenienced or find yourself avoiding the activity, you'll have to work a little harder at getting started. Once you enjoy the physiological benefits, you're more likely to look forward to getting on those walking or running shoes and opening the door to an enjoyable experience. Decide whether or not having a partner will motivate you. Some seem to enjoy the solitude while others enjoy the company of others. The choice depends on your personality or how you spend your typical day.

PROFESSIONAL GROWTH TIP

Before beginning any rigorous plan, consult your physician (especially if you are over the age of 40 and/or have a medical problem).

Walking

If you are moderately overweight, recovering from an injury, or spend your days sitting in class, traveling hours in your car, or working at the computer, walking is probably for you. Don't push yourself too hard. This can cause fatigue or injury and turn you off altogether. Get a good pair of walking shoes and open the door! Choose a speed and duration that you are comfortable with and gradually increase them along with your frequency as you become more fit. Once you've started, the real challenge is sticking with your plan. Here are some of the ways you can stay on course.

- Selftalk along the way. (I can do it! I'm proud of myself for taking action. Look how far I've come.)
- Enjoy the experience. (Take in the fresh air and scenery. Support others along the way.)
- Don't think of it as work.

Think of All the Benefits!

REGULAR WALKING CAN DECREASE:

- Anxiety
- Blood pressure
- Body fat
- Bone loss
- Constipation
- Depression
- Falls and fractures
- Glucose
- Mobility limitations
- Pain
- Risk of some cancers
- Risk of heart attack and stroke
- Risk of diabetes
- Stress
- Weight

(*Source: Arthritis Today,* 2003)

REGULAR WALKING HELPS IMPROVE:

- Aerobic capacity
- Balance
- Blood sugar
- Bone density
- Cartilage and joint health
- Joint mobility
- Life span
- Mental capacity
- Mood
- Muscle mass and tone

- Circulation
- Energy level and endurance
- Flexibility and range of motion
- Heart health

(*Source: Arthritis Today,* 2003)

- Overall general health
- Quality of life and sleep
- Feeling of accomplishment
- Self-esteem

Running

If you think walking is too easy and you're looking for something more challenging, then you may want to try a combination of both. Check your local sporting goods store for a shoe that is made for runners. Over a period of weeks, you will gradually increase your speed and duration while spending less time walking and more time running. For example, during week one you may alternate two minutes of running followed by four minutes of walking. By week number five, you should be able to alternate four minutes of running followed by two minutes of walking. As your running time increases, the repetitions per session should gradually decrease. Both walkers and runners use music to move them as well as to help them keep track of their time to switch from walking to running and back again. When you make progress, reward yourself with a new music CD.

PROFESSIONAL GROWTH TIP

Be sure to do some warmup exercises (stretching or jumping in place) for five minutes before beginning your new routine.

Think of All the Benefits!

- Burns more calories than walking alone
- Builds stronger bones
- Releases your body's endorphins ("runner's high")

- Improves your overall mood
- It's energizing!

Strength Training

Strength training (or weight lifting) is an excellent activity for shaping your body, a benefit that walking or running alone doesn't offer. Strength training is easy, can be done at home, and requires as few as eight minutes each day. Your only investment is a pair of free weights or small dumbbells. Check at your local sporting goods store for a weight that is appropriate for you.

To shape your chest, lie on a mat on your back with your knees bent and your feet flat on the floor. With a dumbbell in each hand, press weights upward as you extend your arms from a starting position of elbows in line with shoulders and forearms at a right angle with your upper arm. Exhale as you press upward and hold for several seconds. Inhale as you return to your starting position. Try to do 10 to 12 repetitions.

Your shoulders can be shaped by standing with your feet shoulder-width apart with dumbbells in your hands as they rest at your side (elbows relaxed). Begin exhaling as you lift the weights away from your side until they are at about your shoulder level. Hold for several seconds and then return to starting position as you inhale.

Strength training exercises can be done *without* dumbbells, using your own body weight. Your own body weight can be used to shape your calves and thighs and tighten abdominal muscles (e.g., squats, leg lifts, crunches). Most fitness magazines feature strength training exercises. Pick up one if the benefits of this activity appeal to you.

Think of All the Benefits!

- Firms your body
- Helps you lose fat without losing muscle
- Less fat means a lower risk of cancer
- Improves your strength
- Makes you feel healthier and look better

Stretching

Stretching is indeed a feel-good activity. We sometimes do it without thinking. Infants do it! Stretching is a very natural activity that leaves you feeling relaxed and refreshed. It requires no special equipment and doesn't take much longer than taking a deep breath.

As we age, our muscles and tendons start to shorten and tighten. You must have seen a elderly person with poor posture associated with these changes. Poor posture can decrease blood flow to vital organs and decrease lung capacity, which further compromises oxygen demands. All of this leaves our body feeling tired and stiff. The good news is flexibility can be restored by stretching regularly. Stretching will also complement your walking or running routine.

It is important to stretch only to the point where you feel (comfortable) tension in the abdominal muscles. If you feel pain, stop! Do each stretch two to five times. Breathe and relax during your routine. Finally, don't bounce.

Think of All the Benefits!

- Relaxes your mind and body
- Relieves muscle and joint pain
- Enhances body awareness and mental focus
- Improves posture
- Improves coordination
- Reduces stiffness
- Improves circulation
- Helps you perform tasks more easily with improved range of motion (ROM)

EMOTIONAL HABITS THAT CREATE A HEALTHY MIND AND BODY

By improving your emotional habits, you can improve your body's physical health. What does this mean? Do you remember how stress-free you felt the last time you had a good laugh, or how peaceful you felt when you first fell in love? These were times that your mind was being very good to your body. Again, it is the increased activity of the feel-good chemicals (dopamine, serotonin, and other euphoric substances) that heightens your sense of overall well-being. Below is a list of some very healthy options. Again, the choice is yours!

- Learn to relax by meditating
- Build friendships
- Do things that a healthy individual would do
- Don't dwell
- Set yourself up for success
- Laugh a lot!

Learn to Relax by Meditating

You cannot afford *not to* learn how to relax. If I say the word *meditation,* are you thinking, That's just not for me? My father would say the same thing; however, he *does* meditate each morning. He spends a few moments in prayer, thankful for all the things he values in life. He doesn't call it meditation. He doesn't have a name for it, he just does it! After 40 years, it comes naturally. Call it what you want, but see what happens when you find a quiet place, close your eyes, and clear your mind.

It takes only five minutes. Find a place where you won't be distracted. Sit with your back straight. Allow your shoulders to drop. Close your eyes, or allow them to rest downward, focusing on nothing. Let your breathing become deep and rhythmic. Aim for 15-minute sessions, twice a day.

Dr. Oz, director of Columbia Presbyterian's Heart Institute, relies on the Eastern technique—meditation—to prepare his patients for surgery and steer them gently toward recovery. His explanation for offering preoperative meditation: "Because it works" (Oz, 2003).

> ## PROFESSIONAL GROWTH TIP
>
> *Studies have shown that meditation can counteract the fight or flight response that floods the body with cortisol.*

Build Friendships

How can friendships reduce stress? Researchers at the University of California at San Francisco report that the "hormone (oxytocin) best known for its role in inducing labor may influence our ability to bond with others" (University of California at San Francisco, 1999). Other studies suggest that befriending may increase the levels of oxytocin present in circulation, countering stress and producing a calming effect. Although this may be more evident in women than in men, study after study proves that belonging to a social group or being in a long-term healthy relationship reduces our risk of disease by lowering blood pressure, heart rate, and cholesterol. Take the time to build friendships. It can help you live a happier and healthier life.

> ## PROFESSIONAL GROWTH TIP
>
> *Maintaining strong friendships is as important as maintaining your health. They are intimately blended.*

Do Things That Healthy Individuals Do

Do you want to be healthy? Act healthy! Do things that healthy individuals do. Resist the temptation to stay indoors when the sun is shining. Limit your time in front of the television. Eat apples and carrots in small quantities until your appetite for fresh produce increases. Take the stairs instead of the elevator. Give meditation or even yoga a try. You will soon feel very much in place with your newly formed healthy habits. After all, you are what you do!

Don't Dwell

Let go of the past. I know it's easier said than done. Letting go takes time, but as you build new friendships, find new ways to spend your time, set personal goals, and resolve to be a better person, you will have no time left for dwelling. So let go. Most people have experiences they would rather not remember. You are not alone. Stand tall, learn to be optimistic, and move on. You will find yourself even more driven as you allow yourself to experience a more positive you.

PROFESSIONAL GROWTH TIP

Each time a negative thought enters your mind, simply say "delete . . . delete" and move on.

Set Yourself Up for Success

We all have our unique talents. Not everyone can be a patient and loving parent. Nor can everyone aspire to be a chemical engineer or skilled plastic surgeon. Examine your values and then be realistic about your career and personal goals. Experts recommend that you set your goals in increments rather than focus on one long-term and lofty goal that is nearly unattainable. When you set unrealistic goals, the journey can be unpleasant as you experience hardships along the way. No, there is no substitute for hard work. But recognize your aptitude before determining your ultimate career or personal objectives. With self-awareness skills, setting your goals should be a success in itself.

Laugh a Lot!

Laughter really does promote physical health. It is my favorite form of emotional workout. I know from personal experience that laughter can improve concentration, self-esteem, and overall well-being. What I *didn't* know until recently was that laughter causes higher regions of the brain to "coordinate a sudden surge in adrenaline and other stress hormones, driving up heart rate, blood pressure, and metabolism while initiating a respiratory response close to hyperventilation." The real reward, says Robert Provine, professor of psychology at the University of Maryland, may have *more* to do with the social bonds that laughter helps strengthen (Selim, 2003, p. 65).

Let's examine the physiological changes that occur during laughter:

- Lungs improve oxygen supply to vital organs.
- Adrenal glands release adrenaline and cortisol.
- Muscles of the abdomen, legs, and back contract, mimicking aerobic exercise.
- Heart rate and blood pressure increase to provide oxygen to muscles, then return to baseline following the outburst.
- Dopamine and other excitatory chemicals are released by the brain, enhancing the feeling of well-being.

If you're still not convinced that laughter is the best medicine, consider this: multiple studies show that higher levels of antibacterial and antiviral cells are found in saliva following an outburst of laughter.

As you face assignment deadlines, overwhelming workloads, and personal responsibilities, look for opportunities to laugh. Laughter's "aftershocks" just might propel you from one difficult assignment to the next. Remember, learning should be a satisfying experience. I believe that laughter is one of the most available forms of stress relief.

PROFESSIONAL GROWTH TIP

You're 30 times more likely to laugh when you're with other people than you are when you are alone.—Robert Provine (Johnson, 2003, p. 66).

So you see that by changing your emotional habits, your body responds by releasing a number of natural pleasure-causing hormones and neurotransmitters. Your mind is doing great things for your body.

It is unfortunate to see a dedicated health care worker who neglects her or his own emotional and physical needs. Promise yourself as you prepare to enter the workforce that you will not rob yourself of a wholesome lifestyle that you are most entitled to. Remember to think happy thoughts, spend time with friends, don't dwell, learn to relax, and laugh. The benefits are too good *not* to give it a try!

Seriously! This is no laughing matter. The immediate onset of psychological and physiological perks will amaze you. Okay, maybe the benefits listed below are something to laugh about.

- A feeling of euphoria
- A calmer body
- A good night's rest
- A feeling of self-control/higher self-esteem
- Increased efficiency of the immune system
- Improved coordination
- Improved concentration
- Reduced risk of heart disease, stroke, diabetes, and infectious diseases

AVOIDING YOUR OWN HEALTH CRISIS

Some "quick-fix" remedies for stress can be your own worst enemy, leaving you even more stressed after the effects wear off. Are any of these habits in your arsenal of stress busters?

- Shift work
- Food binging
- Alcohol abuse
- Cigarette smoking
- Prescription drug misuse
- Ecstasy, heroin, and speed

Shift Work

More than 22 million Americans work evening, rotating, or on-call shifts and face sleep-related problems (American Academy of Sleep Medicine, 2000). People who work shifts force their bodies to sleep at a time when their bodies would normally be awake, thus interfering with the natural (circadian) rhythm that their bodies have come to know. The circadian rhythm is a hormonal rise and fall that helps the body respond to a stressful morning and a busy evening. This hormone, cortisol, rises early in the morning and again in the evening to help when our activity level is the highest. Someone who "picks up" an off-shift (i.e., 11 to 7) will have difficulty falling asleep in the morning, as the cortisol level will be elevated. The worker will feel less relaxed and have more of a get-up-and-go feeling, making it difficult to sleep. This is the same physiological stress one will experience with jetlag (i.e., touching down at 7:00 A.M. local time when your body "knows" that it's 10:00 P.M. and ready for sleep).

What to Do?

Shift workers are continually sleep-deprived. Night shift workers who sleep during the day get an average of two to four hours less sleep than day shift workers (American Academy of Sleep Medicine, 2000). Your work schedule should be one that feels natural to you. Some individuals actually prefer to work evenings and nights, as they feel more awake during those hours. Here is a variety of solutions that should help reduce the stress related to off-shift working hours.

- Take your breaks (and rest) during work hours.
- Keep a regular (day) sleep schedule seven days a week.
- Increase your total hours of sleep time by napping.
- Avoid sleeping pills, as they do not reset your rhythm.
- Avoid caffeine within four hours of your desired bedtime.
- Wear sunglasses on a trip home from the night shift, as the morning sun signals the body to wake up and not go to sleep.
- After a night at work, brush your teeth, shower, put on sleepwear, and make the bedroom comfortable for sleep.

Food Binging

It can be so tempting to eat a huge piece of chocolate cake or down a bag of chips after you've had a stressful day. For some, it might be more of a pattern than an occasional craving. Cravings are often triggered by stress and the foods you crave can be very difficult to resist. A craving is your body's way of telling you that if you go for that piece of chocolate cake or bowl of ice cream, everything will be okay. "But that's not always the case," according to Adam Drewnowski, Ph.D., director of the nutritional-sciences program at the University of Washington. Carbs can trigger the release of serotonin, boosting your mood, but they can also leave you feeling tired and sluggish. This is not a mental state conducive to active learning or critical thinking. Giving in too often can lead to obesity and feelings of helplessness and guilt.

Be prepared for the stress hormones to surge during the school year(s) ahead or any time, for that matter, by having some healthful foods on hand. Here is a grocery list for you:

- Dried fruit
- Nuts
- Energy bars
- Fresh fruits and vegetables
- Cheese
- Healthy shakes
- Natural fruit juices

These food items are perfect substitutes for doughnuts, potato chips, and chocolate candy bars. These items on your *new* grocery list are naturally sweet, high in protein and fiber, and great-tasting. See what trading in candy bars for dried fruits can do for your health and mental well-being.

PROFESSIONAL GROWTH TIP

Caffeine gives you a false sense of energy because it doesn't give your body any real fuel to burn. Coffee and soda are only quick-fixes and should be consumed with a real energy-providing snack.

The American Institute for Cancer Research (AICR) recommends a dinner plate two-thirds filled with plant-based food such as vegetables, fruits, whole grains, and beans and one-third filled with meat, fish, or poultry. You're not only reducing your risk of colon, breast, and prostate cancer, but you're promoting weight loss, a cancer and heart disease fighter in itself.

For more information on weight loss and disease prevention, visit the following Web sites:

- American Heart Association—www.americanheart.org
- American Institute for Cancer Research—www.aicr.org

Alcohol Abuse

It's no secret that the United States is a drinking society. Young people as well as adults are drinking to get drunk every day. But most of these people don't see it as a problem. That's because the thought of being an alcoholic is not easy to swallow. But alcoholism is a disease and it is preventable. Not everyone who drinks (and gets drunk) is an alcoholic. Let's take a look at three types of alcohol use and you decide (honestly) which type, if any, describes your drinking behavior. (1) *Social drinking:* Drinking is done at a slow pace and in moderation and usually at a celebration to lighten the mood or at dinner to stimulate an appetite. (2) *Alcohol misuse:* Drinking leads to inappropriate behavior, aggressiveness, or passing out. For individuals in this category, misuse occurs rarely or infrequently. (3) *Alcohol abuse:* This is drinking taken to the extreme. It is similar to alcohol misuse although alcohol consumption occurs frequently and regularly.

It's a proven fact that scare tactics don't work. During the 1980s elementary school-age children were taught alcohol and drug abstinence. Yet gifted young people require total care at trauma centers across the United States daily from alcohol-related injuries. Some of them will remain paralyzed and unable to eat or talk for the rest of their lives. Alcohol abuse will destroy your personal relationships, prevent you from attaining goals that you once set out to achieve, and, in the end, destroy your nervous system, liver, pancreas, and esophagus (from frequent vomiting and the corrosive effect of liquor).

If you are drinking before school or work, ask yourself: *Why?* If you are drinking alone, using alcohol to get drunk, or seeing your school or work performance starting to slip, it's time to consider that scary thought that you are an alcoholic. If you see these tendencies in yourself, do not wait a day longer to share your concerns with someone that you can trust. Then, allow a professional or a support group such as AA to become involved in your recovery before it's too late.

ALCOHOLICS ANONYMOUS® is a fellowship of men and women who share their experience, strength, and hope with each other that they may solve their common problem.

PROFESSIONAL GROWTH TIP

Accountability for alcohol use, misuse, and abuse begins with each of us.

PROFESSIONAL GROWTH TIP

Plan your next party ahead of time by asking yourself (1) Am I going to drink? *and (2)* How will I do it responsibly?

Cigarette Smoking

"More than 90 percent of patients with lung cancer are, or have been, cigarette smokers. Smoking marijuana increases the risk of cancer for cigarette smokers. Quitting cigarette smoking reduces the incidence of lung cancer" (National Institute of Health, 1997). That is what the U.S. Department of Health and Human Services reports. Yet, cigarette smoking is still on the rise and the age of first-time smokers is becoming younger. Cigarette smoking also increases the risk of heart disease and stroke. If you smoke, talk to your doctor about options for quitting.

Prescription Drug Misuse

Your doctor may prescribe drugs for you that reduce anxiety, tension, panic attacks, or stress. They work by depressing the brain's activity, producing a calming effect. Other drugs might be prescribed for acute pain following surgical procedures or chronic pain associated with injury or disease. Finally, stimulants are occasionally prescribed for younger individuals for attention-deficit hyperactivity disorder or for adults suffering from acute morbid obesity. Whether you are taking antianxiety medication, "pain killers," or stimulants, the precautions are the same. Don't use them with other substances that cause central nervous system depression (alcohol, antihistamines, or over-the-counter cold and allergy medications) and take only as recommended. Long-term use of these prescription drugs can lead to tolerance, physical dependence, withdrawal, or addiction. Talk to your doctor before making any changes to the prescribed instructions on taking the drug.

PROFESSIONAL GROWTH TIP

Don't forget about your body's ability to produce natural pain-relieving, feel-good, and soothing hormones.

Ecstasy, Heroin, and Speed

Those who have experimented with drugs to get high, just once, may soon realize that their habit has escalated to the point where nothing else but getting the drug matters. This can be scary since drug addiction is a burden often carried alone. There are several things you must know before you are faced with the decision to try a drug-induced high (if you haven't already) or before you plan to use your drug of choice again.

- Ecstasy can cause sudden death from a heart attack, seizures, or heat exhaustion. Ecstasy interferes with the brain's ability to absorb serotonin, the body's natural sedative (Werther, 2001).
- Heroin users experience nausea, vomiting, and severe itching, followed by a period of a trancelike state. This mental stupor can last for hours. Repeated use requires more of the drug to get the same feeling. Poor circulation (requiring amputations) and infections (including HIV) are associated with injecting heroin into veins. Due to its effect on the intestinal and urinary systems, heroin can cause chronic constipation and difficulty urinating (Cobb, 2000a).
- Speed stimulates the activity of the brain. Along with the "desired" effect of euphoria (feeling high) an individual can experience irritability or aggressiveness. Long-term use can cause extreme excitability, sleeplessness, anxiety, paranoia, and panic. More serious effects include mental confusion, violent and aggressive outbursts, convulsions, and thoughts of suicide as well as homicide (Cobb, 2000b).

Please visit these Web sites if you or someone close to you uses street drugs.

PROFESSIONAL GROWTH TIP

"Even the healthiest people don't feel happy all of the time"
(Werther, 2001, p. 6).

Center for Substance Abuse Prevention (CSAP)
http://www.samhsa.gov/csap
National Institute on Drug Abuse
http://www.nida.nih.gov

Developing healthy habits takes practice and patience. The consequences of relying on quick fixes, such as recreational drugs, binge drinking, and excessive cigarette smoking as a form of relaxation, can slowly evolve into serious addictions and alcoholism. If you don't smoke, don't start. If you use prescription drugs, use them only as directed. And if you are consuming alcohol or using recreational drugs at school or at the workplace, it is time to get professional help. You may want to start with contacting your school's or employer's health services department.

REFERENCES

American Academy of Sleep Medicine. (2000). *Coping with shift work* [brochure].

Cobb, A. B. (2000a). *Heroin and your veins: The incredibly disgusting story.* New York: The Rosen Publishing Group.

Cobb, A. B. (2000b). *Speed and your brain: The incredibly disgusting story.* New York: The Rosen Publishing Group.

Husseini, N. (2003). *Exercise and depression.* Retrieved March 3, 2003, from http://www.vanderbilt.edu.

Johnson, S. (2003). The brain and emotions. *Discover, 24*(4), 66.

Lemonic, M. D. (2003). A frazzled mind, a weakened body. *Time, 161*(3), 68–69.

National Institute of Health. (1997). *The lungs in health and disease* [brochure].

Oz, M. (2003). Say "om" before surgery. *Time, 161*(3), 71.

Selim, J. (2003). Anatomy of a belly laugh. *Discover, 24*(4), 65.

University of California at San Francisco. (1999, July). *Hormone involved in reproduction may have role in the maintenance of relationships.* Retrieved March 7, 2003, from http://www.oxytocin.org/oxytoc/

Werther, S. P. (2001). *Ecstasy and your heart: The incredibly disgusting story.* New York: The Rosen Publishing Group.

WHERE ARE MY EARNINGS GOING?

Sandra Gaviola

READY FOR NEW VEHICLE?
The Selection Process
Timing
Financing
Auto Insurance
Maintaining Your Car

READY FOR A NEW HOME?
Renting
Buying a New Home

DEBT AND CREDIT COUNSELING

———

In Chapter 1 we discussed the motivational factors that are necessary to keep your spirits high enough to keep you coming back to the classroom day after day. Remember that the most powerful motivational factors are those that are internal or intrinsic in nature. But occasionally we sway toward a more external or extrinsic force and that propels us for a time. Like a pendulum, the forces that move us until graduation day can swing from intrinsic to extrinsic.

It's not unusual to want to purchase new things as soon as you start working. You may be able to purchase some small luxuries or household items with cash, avoiding the credit card crisis that we all fear. However, purchasing some items on credit might be in your best interest for the following reasons: (1) you have the opportunity to start saving cash and (2) you can begin building a good credit rating for future (major) purchases (e.g., auto and home).

———

A BRILLIANT DISCOVERY

The spontaneous spending of cash is a financial problem that sneaks up on the newly employed. They are confident that they will always find the funds and know that credit is almost always available. There is no better time than the present to learn how to manage your money and discover the simple things you can do to establish a savings account and avoid a credit card crisis.

Before consulting a financial planner, prepare a personal financial summary (including the financial information of your partner if he or she is legally or agreeably involved in your money matters). A financial summary is a rundown of two simple lists: total monthly income and total monthly expenditures. If you are spending all of your cash spontaneously, you might be on a slippery slope. Eventually, you may not be able to pay every bill on time or build even a modest savings account. If this sounds familiar, you may be on to something. You may be earning less than you owe, or, spending more than you are earning—a brilliant discovery!

Most financial planners will begin by asking you to describe your thoughts about money. For example, do you see it as a simple tool to acquire practical and necessary items, or do you see it as something different? Do you equate it with self-worth and the power to purchase luxury items, or do you intend to save every possible dollar so that one day you can attain complete financial freedom? Spending habits vary from person to person and say a lot about what you value in life. Have you thought about what you value most in life? Unless you actually see your values in writing, you may never create a financial plan to accomplish your lifelong goals.

Write your eulogy. The purpose of this exercise is to get you thinking about your values, life goals, and how you would most like to be remembered. Dig deep. Think about what you would like to accomplish in your lifetime. This will allow you to focus on the things that are most important to you. If you are a dreamer—and that's what makes us healthy—then dream! Dream big, but don't expect *every* dream to come true. Pare down the list by prioritizing and work toward achieving the goals that you've identified as most important to you.

―――

MONEY ISN'T EVERYTHING

No, money isn't everything until you find yourself sitting at the kitchen table counting quarters. Did you know that *even that* can be avoided? Think about the money that you spent recently. Make a list of every item you purchased this week. Beside each item, write the amount that you spent for it. And finally, circle the items that were not necessary purchases or could have been substituted with less expensive versions or borrowed for free. Add up the amount of money that you could have had on hand at this moment had the circled items never been purchased. This could have been placed into a savings account. Counting change before payday is an overwhelming experience that I sincerely hope you will never have to experience.

PROFESSIONAL GROWTH TIP

Do you have a plan for accomplishing your financial goals? Don't waste any time getting to this very important step in money management.

Depending upon where you are on the educational timeline, the clock may be ticking down to graduation day. This day marks the beginning of two very important events: a new opportunity for full-time employment and an obligation to pay back your student loans. Or did you forget about the *easy money* dispersed in your name? The following section outlines some of the loans that were probably available to you.

EDUCATION LOAN PROGRAMS

Federally subsidized loans are commonly accepted by college students. The U.S. government reports that over $100 billion has been borrowed by students and their families since 1990. Chances are you received a student loan to pay for school. And soon you'll be expected to repay the funds. Although student loans are generally low-interest, you must make every effort to repay on time and according to the terms. This is an excellent way to start building a good credit rating. Below are descriptions of three types of federal student loan programs and ways in which you can avoid problems associated with these loans.

Federal Stafford Loans

This is a federally subsidized loan, which means interest on the loan is paid by the federal government while you are in school and for six months thereafter. This loan is made in your name (the student) only and can be used for expenses related to education (e.g., tuition, books, supplies, and housing). You will receive an amount based upon your financial needs.

Borrowing Limits

In 2003, students attending an undergraduate program (five-year program or less) can borrow a lifetime maximum of $23,000. As you progress through your years of college, the amount you may borrow increases. Check with your financial aid advisor for the most recent data.

Interest Rates

These rates are set annually by the federal government. Since the loans are subsidized by the government, the interest rates are significantly lower than for a general installment loan offered by a bank, credit union, or commercial lender (approximately 3.5 percent). Therefore, most students take advantage of this type of loan program.

Repayment Period

Once you graduate, withdraw, or leave school, you will be granted a six-month grace period. This allows you to adjust to your life changes and also gives you time to prepare for the repayment of your loan debt. During the grace period, your lender will provide you with a repayment disclosure statement containing your repayment terms, including the amount of your monthly payment and the due date of your first payment. Generally, the monthly payment is $50; however, you should talk to your lender to determine other flexible repayment terms that might be available. Payment period can extend up to 10 years.

Start Saving Today

Check with your lender regarding prepaid fees (deducted from your loan proceeds). Ask about *late fees* if you miss a payment.

Federal Perkins Loans

The Perkins loan is also federally funded but distributed as the colleges see fit. Each school receives a predetermined amount of funding each academic year and awards it to students who have high financial needs as defined by the individual school.

Borrowing Limits

In 2003, students attending an undergraduate program can borrow a lifetime maximum of $20,000. Again, the amount you can borrow increases as you progress through your years of college.

Interest Rates

Federal assistance helps keep the interest rates low (approximately 5 percent). Check with your lender for the most recent interest rates.

Repayment Period

Repayment begins nine months after graduating or withdrawing from school. Repayment period may be spread over a 10-year period.

Start Saving Today

If you are just starting out and have little debt or other financial responsibilities, pay more than the monthly minimum on a regular basis. There are late fees if you miss a payment. *Note:* paying down credit card debt that carries a higher interest rate should be your priority.

Federal Parent Loans for Undergraduate Students

Also known as PLUS programs, these loans are available to parents of full-time or half-time dependent undergraduate students. Parents must have an acceptable credit rating in order to qualify. Financial need is not a consideration.

Borrowing Limits

The amount of the loan is limited to the total cost of education, less financial aid received by the student. There is no lifetime maximum.

Interest Rates

This is determined by the federal government as a variable rate. At the time of this publication, it is not to exceed 9 percent.

Repayment Period

Generally, repayment must begin within 60 days after the final loan disbursement for the period of enrollment for which you borrowed. There is no grace period for these loans. This means that interest begins to accumulate at the time the first disbursement is made.

Your parents must begin repaying both principal and interest while you're in school. Under certain circumstances your parents can request a deferment on their loan. Generally, the eligibility for requesting a deferment that applies to Stafford loans also applies to PLUS loans. Your parents will be charged interest during the period of deferment.

CONTROLLING YOUR PERSONAL FINANCES

"What finances?" you ask. Assuming you're not panhandling on campus, you must have some funds available to you. If you are an independent student who is working a part-time job, congratulations on your efforts! If you receive a monthly allowance from home, or your parent(s) or guardians are making monthly payments on your student credit card, be aware of the fact that you may be putting a huge drain on those who are trying to help you. Don't misuse the money or forget that credit is a *high-price loan*. The best way to control your personal finances is by keeping track of where your money is going.

Checking Account

Opening a checking account is one way to keep track of where your money is going. It's also a convenient way to pay routine bills by postal or electronic mail or purchase items spontaneously if you don't have a credit card. As a student, there are a few—but very important—features you will want to have with your new checking account. Select a bank that has a convenient location and hours. Ask about a student checking account that requires no minimum balance with free ATM services. *Caution*: writing a check with nonsufficient funds (NSF) available in your account will cost you about $30. Three *bad* checks on a weekend can cost you your full week's earnings or allowance.

Balance your checkbook on a regular basis. This allows you to resolve any discrepancies. Don't forget to record ATM fees, new check purchases, nonsufficient fund fees, or other charges the bank may add. Keep your checking account padded if possible. You will be grateful if the padding prevents just one check from bouncing.

Savings Account

If you have a large amount of money saved, you might want to put it in a place that you can't easily access to prevent over-spending or in an account that pays interest, such as a savings or passbook account. A savings account can be opened with little money; however, it pays very little interest. Perhaps in the future you will have more available cash and will want to consider money market accounts or certificates of deposit (CDs).

Cash on Hand

Travel with less cash on hand if you spend it too easily. If you need an item "now" from the all-night convenience store, take only enough to purchase that item. Convenience stores are warehouses filled with items that are normally purchased on a spontaneous basis. Keep a small box or an envelope in your "top drawer" for cash receipts. You will know where your money is going and have receipts readily available (for possible deductions) on April 15.

When You Know You're in Trouble

Anyone who has mismanaged money can tell you the warning signs. You might be experiencing them now on a small scale. If your spending habits don't improve, the same problems can affect your ability to purchase and maintain your basic needs or acquire small luxuries in the future. You know that you're in trouble when:

- You borrow money frequently.
- You look for ways to make quick money.
- You often use cash advances to pay your monthly bills.
- You often overdraw on your checking account.
- You pay only the *most important* bills each month.

These signs of trouble are not limited to students. Without a plan, the stress and anxiety associated with poor money management can follow you around like a black cloud long after you've entered the job market.

CREDIT CARDS

A college credit card is a practical tool. It can be used to purchase books, pay for school supplies, or make a housing deposit. College students are bombarded by credit card companies as soon as the college entrance process begins. But, beware! Credit cards come with "traps."

Shop Around

If you are planning to get a card with revolving credit (i.e., Master Card or VISA), find one with the lowest interest rate, ask for a low credit limit, and make regular payments on your balance. Read the terms of the agreement. Companies can lure you in at a low interest rate and then within a minimal timeframe increase it. Examine your statement and the envelope contents regularly so this does not go on without your taking action. If you notice that the interest rate was increased, negotiate with the company and threaten to switch if they don't lower it. Credit card companies are desperate for consumers. If negotiations are not successful, switch and request confirmation that the account was permanently closed. You can destroy the card and never use the line of credit again. If it is not officially closed, you can be categorized in a high-risk group by lenders who see that you have open and available credit at your disposal. For instance, if you apply for an auto loan or home mortgage in the future and the lender discovers four inactive credit cards with a $5,000 limit each in your name, you may be declined because of your means to amass $20,000 in credit card debt. Frank Banfer informs us that "even if you request the account be closed, your credit report will probably read 'ABC Bank—account closed.' A new lender will look at that without knowing whether you closed the account or if the credit card company closed it due to poor payment history. Therefore return it 'registered mail, return receipt requested' with the following letter" (Banfer, 2002, p. 36).

ABC Credit Card Company
111 Main Street
Anycity, NY 11111

Re: Account # 1111 2222 3333 4444

Dear Associate:

I would like to close the above account effective immediately. Please indicate on your records and my credit report that the account was closed per cardholder's request.

I will expect to receive written verification that the account has been closed as per my request.

Thank you in advance,

Your signature

Avoid a Credit Card Crisis

Just say *credit card* and all kinds of ideas come to mind: power to purchase, convenience, and immediate enjoyment. Misuse the credit card and this word will come to mind: *crisis*. Lessons on credit card activity, published in *American Nursing Student,* September/October 2002, are summarized below. Use these steps to keep yourself free of credit card debt.

- Remember that credit is a loan. It's real money that you must repay.
- Go slowly. Get one card with a low limit and use it responsibly.
- Study your card agreement closely.
- Try to pay off your total balance each month.
- Pay on time.
- Set a budget.
- Make your card harder to use if you start getting into trouble, such as using one card to pay off another. Carry it only when you plan to use it.

INCREASING YOUR MONTHLY INCOME

Saving money is a surefire way to increase the amount you have left at the end of the month. But after paying your regular monthly bills, you might be asking the question, "Saving what?" If your current expenses are exceeding your earnings, you may want to consider one of the following ways to increase your monthly income.

- Take advantage of the shortage.
- Promote yourself.
- Capitalize on your personal interests.

Take Advantage of the Shortage

Having health care-related credentials makes you a highly marketable individual today. Cities throughout the United States are underserved by health care professionals. At this time, health care workers are at a

premium. Check the Internet for agencies that arrange travel assignments for individuals who are free to relocate for several months on
the average. The plans may vary among agencies, but the opportunity
to increase your income is guaranteed.

Promote Yourself

Keep up with technology and changes within your profession. Normally, few individuals are self-directed enough to set higher goals
once they've found employment. It takes motivation and passion for
one to continue learning at a steady pace following graduation. Not
everyone aspires to supervisor or management positions. That's good
news for you if you are a self-directed learner. Offer to attend conferences or workshops relating to your profession. Your manager may
recognize these signs of enthusiasm as an opportunity to delegate his
or her work to you in the future.

PROFESSIONAL GROWTH TIP

Self-directed learners open their own doors to opportunities.

Capitalize on Your Personal Interests

Capitalize on the skills or talents you enjoyed prior to your commitment to health care. Paint on a Saturday afternoon. Teach an aerobics
class on a Tuesday night. Or pick up a few hours in retail during
semester or holiday breaks. This breaks the monotony and can be a
win-win situation as you enjoy the comradeship or physical benefits
while increasing your earnings.

READY FOR A NEW VEHICLE?

This can be an exciting time for you at any age. Don't get out the
checkbook just yet. Some research can save you thousands of dollars.
Purchasing the car of your dreams and relying solely on dealership

information are probably the two biggest blunders made by the inexperienced car buyer.

PROFESSIONAL GROWTH TIP

If you allow the dealer to determine your ability to pay for the car of your dreams, you'll pay!

I settled on a car before examining safety features, reliability, fuel efficiency, or the warranty. I even neglected to establish a price range. I was letting the last issue up to the dealer. *After all*, he would work out a monthly plan based on my ability to pay. *He* did, and *I* paid!

The Selection Process

There are many models available today. You probably already narrowed it down to only a few options based upon your needs, income, or personality. An important feature that should be a priority is safety. The National Highway Traffic Safety Administration and the Insurance Institute for Highway Safety conduct crash, restraint, and rollover tests. These ratings can be found on the following Web sites: www.nhtsa.dot.gov and wwwhwysafety.org.

Determining your price range can be a humbling experience: determine how much you can spend and don't go above that amount. If you have no idea how much you can reasonably afford, call your bank or credit union and ask what the going interest rates are for a three- or four-year loan. And then ask them to calculate a monthly payment for a $20,000 purchase, for example. Let your lender know if you plan to put cash down or have another car that you would like to use as a trade-in. This process will help you determine whether you're in the right price range or not.

New or Used?

There are advantages and disadvantages associated with buying a new car as well as a used car. The major advantages to buying *new* are obvious: appearance, factory warranty, it comes equipped with the latest features, and no one has driven it before you. New cars are also covered under your state's lemon laws (ask your state representative for information on these laws). The disadvantages of buying a new care are equally clear. It is a major financial commitment and if your dealer works out a "deal" whereby you pay low monthly payments for a period of five years, you could be running out of car before you reach the fifth year.

Let's look at the advantages and disadvantages of buying a used car. If you look on the Internet or in the classified ads, you'll see that the availability of low-mileage, affordable cars is rising. If you settle for a preowned auto, your monthly payments are sure to be more affordable. Better yet, you can save thousands more on interest if you are paying for the car with cash. But, be careful, dealers offer only limited warranties on second-hand cars and private sellers offer no guarantee on the reliability or longevity of the car. Lenders recommend having the car looked at by your mechanic prior to the purchase. This will require a deposit for taking the car off the lot. Have an agreement with the dealer that the deposit be refunded if it doesn't pass your mechanic's approval. If a private seller tells you how well the car was maintained while in his or her name, ask to see the written receipts. And, regardless whether you are buying new or used, take along someone who knows more about cars than you do.

Negotiating

You should be familiar with all of the items included in the *sticker price.* First, you will find the manufacturer's suggested retail price, or MSRP. Remember, this is a *suggested* price. Next, expect to see a destination charge. This is the amount the dealer pays to the manufacturer for shipping. And then you will find add-on fees for special features that come standard on the vehicle (manufacturer-installed). Finally, the dealer will probably add on a few hundred dollars for rust proofing or special finish features. The bottom line is the amount the dealer would like you to pay. This is known as the *dealer sticker price.* Whatever that figure is, Tere Drenth, author of *Buying and Leasing a Car,* warns "don't even think of paying it." The dealer sticker price is "equivalent to a price tag on an antique dresser at a flea market: it's just a starting point" (Drenth, 2002).

You won't be prepared to negotiate unless you know what the dealer paid for the vehicle that you want. The dealer would like you to believe that the invoice price listed on the sticker is what the dealership actually paid for the car. What most people don't know is that the manufacturer provides incentives to dealerships in the form of a 2 to 3 percent discount off the MSRP, which means you can pay less than the invoice price and the dealer still makes a profit (Drenth, 2002). Check out the Kelley Blue Book site at www.kbb.com for the MSRP and dealer cost of the vehicle you want. Other *specials* that Drenth advises us to watch for are the cash back and financing specials. The first is simply a cash rebate paid to you from the manufacturer for purchasing its vehicle. It may be around $500 to $1,000. Financing specials are an offer of a lower-end finance rate. This is an *either-or* special, so do the math with the help of someone who is money-savvy to see which of the two will save you more money.

Remember those factory-installed features that increased the price of the car? Do you really need them? Did you plan on buying a car that was loaded with some of the latest features? Maybe you would prefer a more affordable version. Let the dealer know that you *really* like the vehicle but are considering ordering the less-loaded version directly from the manufacturer. The salesperson might throw in the added features for a minimal fee or no fee rather than lose the sale (especially if the vehicle has been sitting on the lot for months).

If possible, start looking for your vehicle before you actually need it. This will give you time to shop around for better deals. If you show a sense of urgency in the showroom, the salesperson will pick up on that and move quickly. He or she may even invite the manager to convince you that you're getting a great car at a great price. If you had any bargaining power, you lost it when they discovered your immediate need to drive off with a new vehicle.

Also, allow some time to compare finance rates offered by your local bank or credit union. Remember, you are not under any obligation to use the dealership's financing program. It may be convenient, but dealers can increase their finance rates and this can translate into thousands of additional dollars over a five-year period. (See *Financing.*)

You will want to have as much pricing information before shopping for a *used* vehicle as you would if you were planning to purchase a new vehicle. Have the following information before comparing prices: the model, year, total mileage, and the overall condition. This is not a science, so expect some variations in the suggested prices. Below is a list of sources along with their Internet sites.

- Kelley Blue Book used-car prices: www.kbb.com
- Auto trader used-car information: www.autoconnect.com
- Pace price guides: www.carprice.com

Trade-ins

Be cautious with a trade-in type negotiation. New car dealers aren't especially interested in buying old cars. You may be told you are getting $3,000 on your trade-in, but the dealer can "make" that a much lower figure with some of his or her clever calculations. Experienced buyers suggest that you check the Kelley Blue Book for your car's value and try to sell it yourself. If, however, you can't sell it and you opt to use it as a trade-in on your new purchase, be sure that the dealer is applying the value of the used car to the new vehicle. This will save you money on sales tax.

Timing

In the automotive sales world, timing isn't everything but it can affect the dealer's need to sell. And, that's a good time for you. So when is it? There are several events (listed below) that influence the dealer's eagerness to move cars off the lot. Watch for ads in your local newspaper, browse the Internet, and look for the manufacturer's national

TV commercials. Buyer-savvy people know how to take advantage of the following events.

- When the new models arrive, last year's models must go.
- End-of-the-month goals put pressure on the sales department.
- Dealers pay tax on inventory once a year. Counting fewer cars on the lot means less inventory tax for the dealership. This is a limited-time offer.

Financing

Although the dealership can set up a finance plan (assuming your application is approved) in just a short time, you should shop around for the best rates first. Your dealership can raise the interest rate by 1 to 2 percent to offset the make up for the "deal" that you got on the car. Compare interest rates on auto loans offered by your local bank, credit union, or even on the Internet before agreeing to finance with the dealership. Apply as much cash down as you are able. This will result in lower monthly payments and a lower finance rate if the balance of the loan can be paid off in three versus five years, for example.

Auto Insurance

Calculation, tables, formulas, and statistics—that's what the auto insurance industry is all about. So consider the following factors before making your final decision on an auto purchase. The cost of insurance can be hundreds of dollars a month and should be researched almost as thoroughly as the purchase of the vehicle itself.

Stereotyping

Auto insurance premiums are calculated not only on *your* personal driving and financial history, but on the reputation of the car itself and the reputation of previous drivers. You can be stereotyped into a premium that you cannot afford by purchasing a car that is not only appealing to you, but popular with thieves and lead-footed drivers. Remember, all cars come with statistics (good and bad). A link to a Web site that you will find helpful when budgeting the cost of auto insurance is https://www.gaininsurance.org/CONSUMER/autorate.asp.

The Age Factor

You have no control over one other factor that affects your auto insurance rates. And that factor is your age. Rates are higher for a younger, less-experienced driver who is generally on the go. At about the age of 25 (assuming you have a "clean" driving record), the cost of auto insurance will start to decline. And, between the ages of 50 to 70 (again, assuming your record is good), you will see your best rates.

You may have no control over your age; however, insurance companies honor programs that statistically classify you as a low risk. For example, insurance agencies offer discounts to new drivers who present a certificate that declares he or she has attended a state-approved driver's training course. These courses are usually offered at a small cost to students at their high school. Drivers who are attending college can have their rates reduced by showing proof of good grades. This is a good student discount. And, individuals who are approaching their mid-50s can attend a safe driver or refresher-type course to reduce their rates.

Take Charge and Save Money

Below is a list of ways you can earn even better rates.

- Buy with cash. Having no loan or lien associated with your vehicle will reduce your insurance needs.
- Opt for a higher deductible ($500).
- Select a car with a good track record. Check the ratings.
- Avoid speeding and obey other traffic laws.
- Never drink alcohol while operating a vehicle.
- Never drink alcohol under the legal age enforced by your state.

A poor credit rating, in general, will classify you as a "moral risk" in the auto insurance industry. This can be translated as follows: one who is in financial straits is statistically more likely to "create" ways to collect on an insurance policy (i.e., fraud). The price of a poor credit rating can be staggering.

Your agent will calculate the cost of your auto insurance based on your past driving record and the features of the vehicle. Information regarding your driving record is made available to your agent through your state's department of motor vehicles. Safety features of vehicles manufactured since 1994 are available on the Internet. No stone is left unturned by the agency when determining the cost of your auto insurance.

PROFESSIONAL GROWTH TIP

If convicted of a DUI, the cost of auto insurance may not be the only concern one might have. A number of companies will not even accept a new driver with a DUI.

Maintaining Your Car

If your car is not maintained because you're too busy with your schoolwork to worry about those fast food wrappers, coffee cups, and papers on the floor, then you're forgiven. But, when you make your first serious purchase, get serious about the maintenance. Have tires rotated regularly and replace bald tires. Have your oil and air filter changed as recommended. See a mechanic as soon as you notice a difference in the performance or an unusual noise. Small problems can become big expenses.

READY FOR A NEW HOME?

Whether you are going to rent or buy largely depends on your financial and personal status. If you are just beginning, you will need some time to save sufficient funds for a down payment and the closing costs that come with buying. And, you might want to wait until you are more established at your job and feel that you and your new town or city are a good fit. Until then, renting is probably the better option.

Renting

Renting is smart way to begin your independent lifestyle. You are free of most maintenance and able to relocate on a relatively short notice (an advantage over the home owner). Normally, your landlord will expect a security deposit (equal to one month's rent) along with the first month's rent on the day you move in. Typically rent is due on the first day of the month. Common courtesy and timely payment will go a long way in satisfying the landlord and avoiding costly legal fees. Before moving in, get the agreement in writing. This is called a *lease*. Be certain all of the parties moving in are involved in the legal agreement (e.g., a $500 rental fee should be divided equally between two occupants, with a separate lease prepared in the amount of $250 per individual). Be sure that you and the other occupant(s) have agreed (in writing) on the method of monthly utility payment. All agreements should be signed by the parties involved and dated. Finally, you may want to discuss refrigerator rules, or who is responsible for purchasing day-to-day household supplies. This can be done by assigning certain rooms (i.e., a kitchenette or bathroom supplies). These guidelines are useful in a dorm setting as well.

PROFESSIONAL GROWTH TIP

Consider your eating habits and financial status when selecting a college meal plan. Most campus eateries have convenient and late hours, making this a more sound choice. Having dinner at a public restaurant (to break the monotony) is a good idea, but don't forget about the cost of drinks and of course a 15 percent tip.

PROFESSIONAL GROWTH TIP

Even good friends should enter into a legal agreement as this is more likely to prevent, rather than cause, a falling-out in the future.

Below is a list of questions that often go unasked until it's too late. Address your questions and request that your landlord clarifies the conditions in writing on the agreement before you sign.

- What (precisely) is included in the cost of rent (e.g., appliances, trash removal, utilities, cable)?
- If I improve the condition of the apartment/house, will the monthly rent be adjusted?
- Who is responsible for lawn care or snow removal?
- May I have extended guests or pets?
- Is off-street parking available?
- Who should I call in the event of appliance or utility failure?
- May I call 24-7?

Ideally, you will establish a good relationship with your landlord and never need legal advice. You should note that renters' rights vary from state to state (and won't be included in this section). Please check your state's renter's laws or ask an attorney or your state representative for more information. You can avoid most legal issues by following these guidelines:

- Always pay the rent on time.
- Notify the landlord of appliance or utility failure as soon as possible.
- Keep the premises neat and clean.
- Avoid excessive traffic in and out of the apartment.
- Notify the landlord of long-term travel plans.
- Request that you be present if repairs or inspections need to be made.

Buying a New Home

Oh, the joy of buying a new home! Just one walk-through and you're thinking, "I could work a second job to afford this home." If you're thinking along those lines, you are probably looking at homes out of your price range. But, how do you really know what you can afford? The cost of the home is just a starting point. The additional professional service and application fees listed below can add thousands more to the purchase price.

- Loan application fee
- Loan originating fee
- Appraisal fee
- Credit report fee
- Lender's inspection fee
- Document preparation fee
- Title search fee
- Settlement or closing fee

This section will show you how to establish your price range and outline common mistakes made by first-time home buyers.

Knowing What You Can Afford

Often, the first person you contact when you are interested in buying a home is a real estate agent. Although they can be very helpful in finding the home of your choice, "they may serve the interests of the seller, and not your interests as the buyer" (U.S. Department of Housing and Urban Development, 2002). This can result in your paying more for the home than at what it is valued or borrowing more than you can afford to pay on a monthly basis. For these reasons, you would be wise to consult a local bank or credit union. Gather records that will enable the lender to compare your assets with your liabilities (e.g., tax returns, credit card debt, regular monthly expenses, savings accounts, and proof of equity in existing real estate). As a general rule, "your monthly house payments (mortgage payments, taxes, and insurance) should not exceed 28 percent of your gross (pretax) monthly income. Your total monthly debt payments (house, credit card, student loans, and other debts) should not exceed 35 percent" (Lloyd, 2002, p. 250). Ask your lender about short-term loans with low interest rates versus long-term loans and higher interest rates. For more on how much you can afford, see the following sources or their Web sites.

- HSH Associates—www.hsh.com
- Bank Rate Monitor—www.bankrate.com
- Quicken's Mortgage information— www.quickenmortgage.com

PROFESSIONAL GROWTH TIP

Determine with your lender how much home you can afford before calling on a real estate agent.

Once your price range is established, don't exceed that amount and *never* tell the agent how much you are willing to pay for a home. Experts advise us against divulging too much information in general to the real estate agent, including how much you *really want* the home. This is bound to reduce your negotiating power. Finally, don't fall into common real estate schemes that place an excessive amount of pressure upon you. The following are common examples:

- The real estate agent states she is planning to show the same property to her "son" or another close relative in the very near future.
- You receive a phone call from the real estate agent just 24 hours after a second walkthrough. She states that two offers were made by other individuals and that you should act quickly if you are really interested.
- Your real estate agent advises you to make an offer near the asking price so that you don't lose it to another family.

Home-Buying Mistakes

It's easy to make home-buying mistakes. Often we are so involved with our professional and personal lives that we unwittingly place our personal finances in the hands of unprincipled sellers. Use the following guidelines to avoid home-buying mistakes.

- Don't disclose anything to your agent that will decrease your negotiating power.
- Stop dealing with an agent if you discover misrepresentation.
- Request a contract "out." This allows you to void the buyer/seller contract if you discover (within a specified period of time) that costly repairs are needed or you can't get suitable financing.
- Hire an independent inspector.
- Keep a deposit on the home to no more than 10 percent of your offer price.
- Have an independent lawyer review the contract before signing.
- Don't buy the best house in a poorly kept neighborhood. In terms of resale value, it's better to buy a modest house in a better neighborhood.

Don't forget, lenders are very competitive today. Don't sign a loan agreement without negotiating or comparing rates and terms with those offered by other institutions. This is probably one of the largest purchases you ever make. Taking the steps necessary to get the most for your money will allow you to feel confident when it is time to sign the mortgage loan agreement.

DEBT AND CREDIT COUNSELING

There are a number of debt/credit counseling firms available. Most are run as nonprofit organizations. You will be asked to make a list of all creditors, expenses, and sources of income. The firm will then negotiate a payment schedule with your creditors. You will have to make a portion of your income available to them to satisfy those obligations on a weekly basis. "If you renege or you're late, your account can be turned over to a collection agency. Rarely is there a second chance" (Banfer, 2002, p. 36).

No one wants to think about the filing of bankruptcy, but there are times when no other options are available. There are basically two avenues under bankruptcy proceedings: liquidation and reorganization. The proceedings are described below.

- Chapter 7—Liquidation. All nonexempt assets are distributed to the creditors and the balance of the obligations is forgiven.
- Chapter 11—Reorganization. Debtor keeps and operates the business and establishes a repayment plan for the creditors.
- Chapter 12—Adjustment of debts of a family farm with regular income.
- Chapter 13—Adjustment of debts of an individual with regular income.

_____

REFERENCES

Avoiding credit card crisis. (2002). *American Nursing Student, 4*(1), 21.

Banfer, F. A. (2002). *The no b.s. guide to getting the most from your money.* Johnstown, PA: Asset Planning Publishing.

Lloyd, N. (2002). *Simple money solutions: 10 ways you can stop feeling overwhelmed by money and start making it work for you.* New York: Times Business.

Drenth, T. (2002). *Fastread: Buying and leasing a car.* Avon, MA: Avon Media Corporation.

U.S. Department of Housing and Urban Development. (2002). *Buying your home: Settlement costs and helpful information* [Brochure]. Washington, DC.

COMMON PROOFREADER MARKS

Operational Signs

℮	Delete
⊃	Close up; delete space
℮	Delete and close up (use only when deleting letters within a word)
Stet	Let it stand
∧#	Insert space
¶	Begin new paragraph
⊐	Move right
⊏	Move left
⊐⊏	Center
⊓	Move up
⊔	Move down
FL	Flush left
FR	Flush right
‖	Align vertically
∩	Transpose
SP	Spell out

Typographical Signs

ital	Set in italic type
(Rom)	Set in roman type
bold	Set in boldface type
/c	Set in lowercase
CAPS	Set in capital letters
SC	Set in small capitals
(wf)	Wrong font; set in correct type
∧	Insert here or make subscript
∨	Insert here or make superscript

Punctuation Marks

∧	Insert comma
∨	Insert apostrophe or single quotation mark
∨ ∨	Insert quotation marks
⊙	Insert period
⑦	Insert question mark
⊙	Insert semicolon
⊙	Insert colon
=	Insert hyphen
{ }	Insert parentheses

INDEX

adrenaline, 172
Alcoholics Anonymous (AA), 188
American Institute for Cancer Research
    (AICR), 187
*Associated Press Stylebook and Libel
    Manual*, 53

behavior. *See* professional appearance
    and behavior
Buying and Leasing a Car (Drenth), 207

Career Success for Health Care Profes-
    sionals Video Series, vii—viii
Chicago Manual of Style, 52–53
Child Abuse Prevention and Treatment
    Act, 167
classrooms, 20–21
  classroom interaction, 27–28
clinical environment, the, 44
  and clinical evaluation, 47
  learning from, 46
  patient care considerations, 46–47
  and performance standards, 45–46
  and professional behavior, 44–45
Complete Works of Winnie the Pooh
    (Milne), 52
cortisol, 172–73

Doing Work You Love (Gilman), 120
dopamine, 174, 180

Drenth, Tere, 207
Drewnowski, Adam, 186

emotional intelligence (EI), 76–77
endorphins, 174
enthusiasm, 111
  and choosing the wrong program,
    114–15
  and the demands of higher educa-
    tion, 111–12
  dwindling, 112
    reasons for, 113–14
    what to do about, 114–21
  generating, 128–33
  lack of in the workplace, 125–26
    reasons for, 126–28
  maintaining, 121–25

Farber, Barry, 125
financial health, 194–95
  controlling personal finances,
    199–200
    cash, 200–201
    checking accounts, 200
    recognizing trouble, 201
    savings accounts, 200
  credit cards, 201
    avoiding credit card crisis, 203
    shopping for, 201–2
  debt and credit counseling, 216–17